Artsy Fartsy

Cultural History of the Fart
Volume One

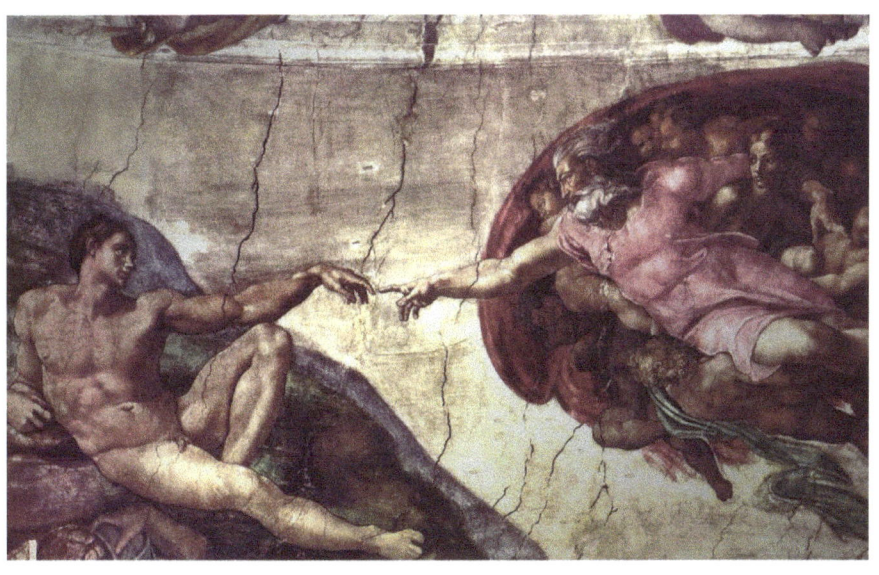

Joseph B. Weiss, MD, FACP, FACG, AGAF
Clinical Professor of Medicine,
Gastroenterology
University of California, San Diego

Artsy Fartsy: Cultural History of the Fart Volume One

Copyright © 2016 Joseph B. Weiss, MD
   SmartAsk Books
   Rancho Santa Fe, California, USA
   www.smartaskbooks.com

ISBN-13: 978-1-943760-16-9 Volume One
ISBN-13: 978-1-943760-17-6 Volume Two
ISBN-13: 978-1-943760-03-9 Combined Volumes

All rights reserved. No part of the text of this book may be reproduced, reused, republished, or retransmitted in any form, or stored in a database or retrieval system, without written permission of the publisher.

Last digit is the print number: 9 8 7 6 5 4 3

Artsy Fartsy: Cultural History of the Fart Volume One

Dedication

This volume is dedicated to clearing the air of the misperception that a fart is anything other than a normal physiologic process common to all humanity. Nature and natural processes should be universally accepted as one of the cherished principles of basic human rights.

I am indebted to my loved ones, Nancy, Danielle, Jeremy, Courie, Lizzy & Indy who have offered their insights, suggestions, comments, and unwavering support throughout the long process of having this project finally come to pass. You will always be the mighty wind beneath my wings.

Artsy Fartsy: Cultural History of the Fart   Volume One

I. **Table of Contents**

II. **Preface**   VIII

III. **Introduction**   1

IV. **Etymology - Origin of the Word Fart**   4

V. **Physiology - Digestion and the Fart**   7

VI. **Chronology of Fart in the Arts**   21
    Hieronymus Bosch
    Michelangelo di Lodovico Buonarroti Simoni
    Pieter Bruegel the Elder
    Medieval Manuscripts
    Francisco Goya
    Wolfgang Amadeus Mozart
    James Gillray
    Louis-Léopold Boilly
    Richard Newton
    Japanese Lithographs Edo Period
    Utagawa Kuniyoshi
    George Cruikshank
    S. Stoutshanks
    Richard Wagner
    Aubrey Beardsley
    Joseph Pujol (Le Pétomane)
    James Ensor
    Canadian Broadcast Corporation
    Salvador Dali
    Cinematic Arts
    Bollywood Hindi Movies
    Seinfeld
    Mr. Methane
    Budweiser Super Bowl Commercial
    The Lion King
    Cartoonists
    Children's Book Art
    The Simpsons
    Family Guy
    South Park
    Beavis & Butt-Head
    Chen Wenlin
    Ontario Ministry of Health
    Advertising & Marketing

VII. **Chronology of Fart in History**   82

Artsy Fartsy: Cultural History of the Fart Volume One

Bel-Phegor
Bible Prophets
Pythagoras
Herodotus
Hippocrates
Aristotle
Metrocles
Cicero
Claudius
Seneca
Flavius Josephus
Plutarch
Babylonian Talmud
Elagabalus
Whoopee Cushion
Yoga
St. Jerome
Augustine of Hippo (St. Augustine)
Islam Hadith
Sir Thomas Moore
Desiderius Erasmus
Martin Luther
HRH Queen Elizabeth I
Michel de Montaigne
Henry Ludlow
Oliver Cromwell
Lord John Wilmot, Earl of Rochester
Benjamin Franklin
Thomas Blount
Immanuel Kant
Charles James Fox
Abraham Lincoln
Sir Richard Burton
John Gregory Bourke
Sigmund Freud
T.E. Lawrence of Arabia
Sir Winston Churchill
Adolf Hitler
Josef Stalin
Sir Robert Hutchinson
Charles de Gaulle
Lyndon Baines Johnson
Ronald Reagan
H.M. Queen Elizabeth II
George W. Bush
Muammar Gaddafi
H.H. the 14th Dalai Lama of Tibet

Artsy Fartsy: Cultural History of the Fart Volume One

Global Warming

VIII. Chronology of Fart in Literature (Volume Two)

Bel-Phegor
Aristophanes
Petronius
Marcus Valerius Martialis
Arabian Nights
Dante Alighieri
Rutebeuf
William Langland
Geoffrey Chaucer
François Rabelais
John Heywood
William Shakespeare
Francois Béroalde de Verville
Ben Jonson
John Donne
Sir John Suckling
John Milton
John Aubrey
Daniel Defoe
Lord John Wilmot Earl of Rochester
Jonathon Swift
Voltaire
Henry Fielding
Jean Anthelme Brillat-Savarin
William Blake
Johann Wolfgang Von Goethe
Jacques Collin de Plancy
Honoré de Balzac
Victor Hugo
Edward Lear
Charles Pierre Baudelaire
Gustave Flaubert
Sir Richard Burton
Samuel Clemens (Mark Twain)
Émile Zola
James Joyce
D. H. Lawrence
Aldous Huxley
Henry Miller
Ernest Hemingway
Thomas Wolfe
W.H. Auden
Roald Dahl

Samuel Beckett
J.D. Salinger
Kurt Vonnegut, Jr.
Norman Mailer
William Styron
George MacDonald Fraser
John Barth
John Kennedy Toole
Philip Roth
George Carlin
Sir Salman Rushdie
James Patterson
Iain Banks
Howard Stern
Melina Marchetta
Children's Books

IX. **Colloquialism, Idiom, & Synonym of Fart**   170

X. **Fart in Foreign Languages**   182

XI. **Afterword**   185

XII. **Index**   189

Artsy Fartsy: Cultural History of the Fart Volume One

II. Preface

The book provides an entertaining overview of the fart in human culture and history, not an extensively referenced academic treatise. I expect that many will be surprised that the fart was a subject near to the hearts and minds of many illustrious and enlightened notables over the course of thousands of years of human history. The cultural mores of Western society have evolved and the fart has become a normal physiological event that has become more tolerated, although not yet universally accepted. Although the fart in human history has more than enough cultural value, I included some of the wisdom and maxims of the notables quoted to further enlighten the reader. It is my hope that **Artsy Fartsy, Cultural History of the Fart** is not only an informative and entertaining volume, but that the included content on digestion enhances the health and wellness of the reader. Hopefully, the reader will be stimulated to learn about their health and wellness in general, and about the digestive process in particular, as they read the subsequent entry on the origins of fart.

What is a fart, but a puff of nothingness, a wind of air? It is a weight so slight as to be immeasurable, a volume that can be compressed to fit on a pinhead. It can escape detection by stealth and silence, with odor so subtle as to be undetectable. It can give joyous pleasure and comfort to the one who releases it, and offence hostility, or amusement in others if detected. Of course, it can also grow in volume and intensity of sound and odor to magnify its presence to the point of being overwhelming. Even the word itself is a party to this paradox. How many words that describe a wind that can be so subtle and innocuous, find them banned from public discourse. The censorship of the word has played a role in modifying our literary heritage. Perhaps the passage in Shakespeare's *Romeo and Juliet*: "What's in a name? That which we call a rose, by any other name, would smell as sweet." was originally submitted as: "What's in a name? That which we call a fart, by any other name, would smell as tart." This volume is an anthology of human culture from the perspective of a small wind of nothingness. From nothing, the story of the fart in human culture magically expands its sphere of influence to virtually everything. Art, literature, music, science, medicine, cuisine, language, psychology, sociology, philosophy, humor, politics, are just a few of the disciplines that have been influenced by the fart. It has influenced individuals and society, from tyrants to saints, royalty to peasants, polymaths to fools.

In addition to providing an in depth overview of the fart in human culture, this volume also offers a selection of the non-fart wisdom and insights of the cultural illuminati who have contributed to the fart in the arts. The reader will hopefully enjoy and benefit from learning a great deal more about the nothingness of the fart, and the wisdom and culture of something more. As an author of a work of nonfiction, the primary purpose is to inform, educate, and entertain. On another level, the volume is also an allegorical tale about the limits imposed by culture and society on matters that arise in the world of nature outside of human control. It should come as no surprise that some of our greatest cultural works were considered both the apogee and zenith of the arts, with only the judgment of the times in which they were viewed discriminating between condemnation and accolades.

Many historical figures of note were branded heretics, tortured, and martyred only to be canonized and acclaimed saints and genius in later ages. The reverse is also true where celebrated leaders and thinkers have been exposed as charlatans and tyrants. So it best to suspend judgment and let the facts speak for themselves. Determine for yourself whether the fart is innocent and to be freely released, or is guilty and should be confined to the purgatory of the bowels of history.

III. Introduction

Artsy Fartsy, Cultural History of the Fart is a fascinating and factually correct review of the common fart through human culture and history. The cough, sneeze, hiccup, stomach rumble, burp, belch, and other bodily sounds simply cannot compete with the notoriety of the fart. Whether encountered live and in person or through the medium of literature, television, film, art, or music it may leave a powerful and lingering memory. The intent of this volume is to demonstrate that the ubiquitous fart has a more illustrious story to share than just lowbrow humor. The societal standards and cultural acceptance of this normal physiologic event have evolved over the years, and it is currently popular as a point of humor even in sophisticated circles.

To 'Air' is Human, Everything You Ever Wanted to Know About Intestinal Gas covers everything you ever wanted to know about the burp, belch, bloat, fart and everything digestive, but were either too afraid or too embarrassed to ask. Intestinal gas has been produced and released by virtually every human who has ever lived, yet very few people have been provided with the knowledge that can offer comfort and relief. This volume is overflowing with practical information, fascinating facts, surprising trivia, and tasteful humorous insight about this universal phenomenon.

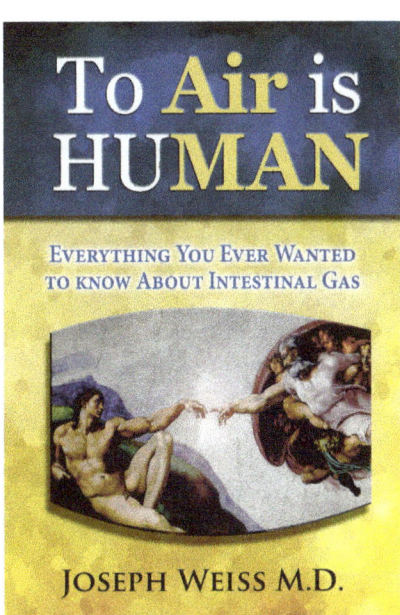 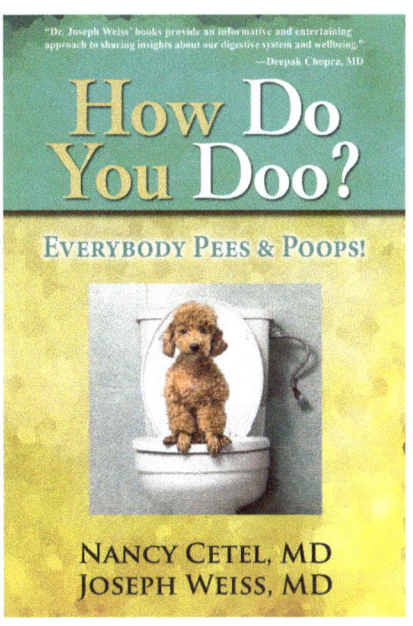

How Do You Doo? Everybody Pees & Poops! A delightfully informative, entertaining, and colorfully illustrated volume with valuable practical insights on toilet training. Tasteful color photographs of animals answering the call of nature allows the child to understand that everybody does it! Additional informative relevant content to entertain the adult while the child is 'on the potty' is included.

The Scoop on Poop! Flush with Knowledge is a uniquely informative tastefully entertaining, and well-illustrated volume that is full of it! The 'it' being a comprehensive and knowledgeable overview of all topics related to the remains of the digestive process. Whether you call it poop, feces, excrement, manure, dung, or the hundred plus other euphemisms, shit happens, and it happens a lot! Tens of billions of pounds and kilograms of it or deposited every day by while diversity of animal and microbial life. Humans alone contribute over three billion pounds a day, and only a small percentage of that is treated by a sewage system

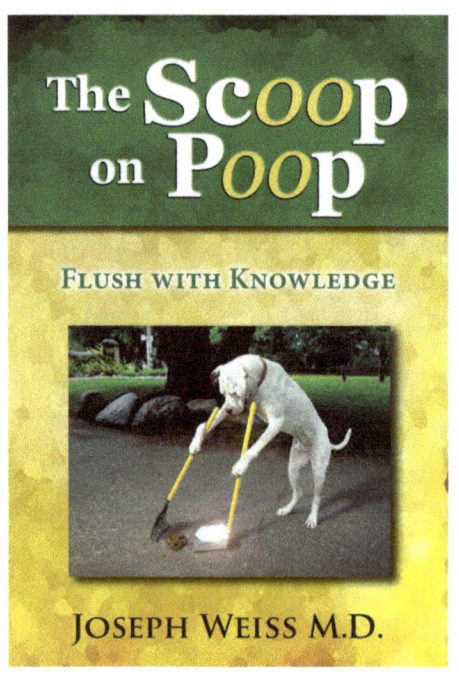 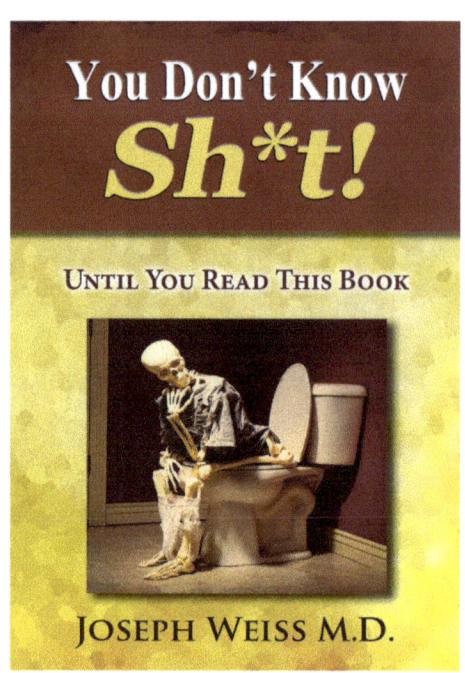

The identical content of The Scoop on Poop has been provocatively and cheekily retitled as ***You Don't Know Sh*t! Until You Read This Book***. This volume is an informative, entertaining and colorfully illustrated fountain of knowledge that is full of valuable information, including eccentricities and peculiarities, about the remains of the digestive process. Although this end result is politely described as feces or excrement, it is more commonly known by one of oldest words in the English language, shit. The book covers everything you ever wanted to know about this subject. Whether you disdain it, or appreciate it, it is part of the human (and animal) experience. The purpose of this volume is to share rarely discussed but very important knowledge about poop. The information ranges from the potentially life-saving to the sidesplitting descriptions of the eccentricities and peculiarities of human behavior on the subject matter. The wealth of information and trivia can sustain a long social conversation, or cut it short abruptly!

AirVeda: Ancient & New Medical Wisdom, Digestion & Gas covers the remarkable advances in the understanding of digestive health and wellness. New information about the critical role of genomics, epigenetics, the gut microbiome, and the gut-brain-microbiome-diet axis are opening new avenues to optimal whole body health and wellness. An appreciation of the ancient wisdom of Ayurveda and other disciplines shows that they had advanced insights into the nature of the human body and the holistic approach. Although intestinal gas, basic bodily functions, and feces have been topics culturally suppressed, knowledge and understanding are needed to achieve and maintain optimal health. This volume, and others in the series, provide an informative and entertaining in depth look at the amazing world of human health and digestion.

"Ayurveda is a 5,000 year old system of natural healing that reminds us that health is the balanced and dynamic integration between our environment, body, mind and spirit. In Dr. Joseph Weiss' book, AirVeda, he provides an informative and entertaining approach to sharing insights about our digestive system and wellbeing by applying the ancient wisdom of Ayurveda to everyday life." **Deepak Chopra, MD**

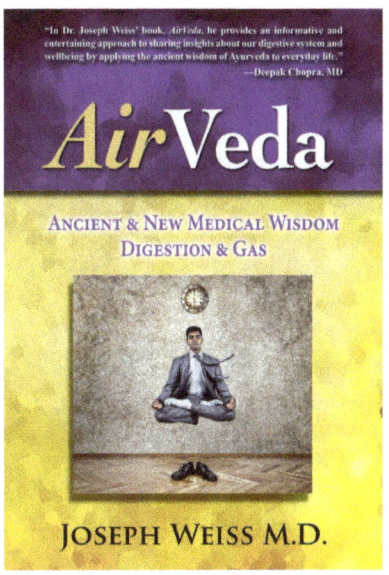 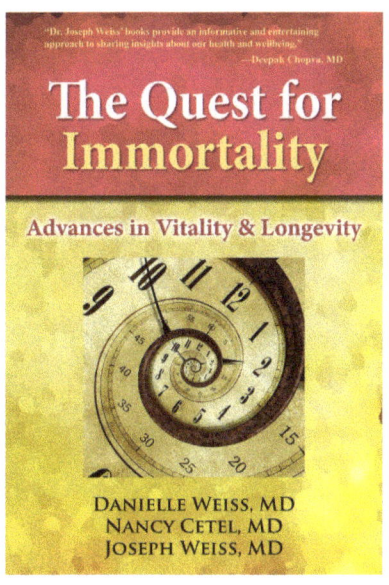

The Quest for Immortality, Advances in Vitality & Longevity provides an informative and enlightening overview of the remarkable advances in science and medicine that are dramatically enhancing human health and lifespan. The volume is written in clear, understandable, and engaging language with striking colorful illustrations. From groundbreaking nanotechnology to genomics and stem cells, the secrets of vitality and longevity are being uncovered along with more traditional advances and practical insights into disease prevention and health enhancement. The website www.smartaskbooks.com has a complete listing of books and programs by Joseph Weiss, MD, FACP, FACG, AGAF, Clinical Professor of Medicine (Gastroenterology), University of California, San Diego.

IV Etymology - Origin of the Word Fart

English is the richest language on the planet, with more words by far than any other. This is due to the significant influence of its history of foreign invasion and occupation, especially during the days of the Roman Empire. Unlike other conquerors, the Romans did not impose the Latin language on the inhabitants of the British Isles. The population adapted their own native tongue to include words borrowed from occupiers and foreign influences to rapidly expand the English vocabulary.

The word fart is the correct word to use in the English language, and indeed is one of its oldest words. The alternative words used, such as flatus and flatulence are not originally English words as they have been borrowed from the Latin, where their general meaning is of a wind or a blowing.

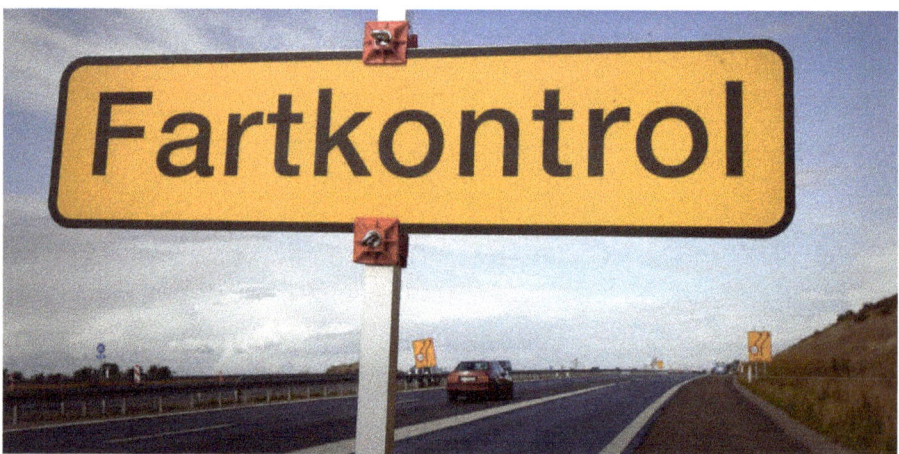

Traffic sign in Sweden, Public Domain

There is controversy as to the derivation of the word fart. It is thought to have Indo-European roots in the Germanic language word farzen. The word fart may have originated as onomatopoeia, a word that phonetically imitates the sound of the event it describes. Another thought is that it was related to the term for partridge, as the bird makes a similar sound when it is disturbed in its natural habitat and takes flight. How it made that transition may be an enlightening example of the evolution of words and language.

The Indo-European word *perd* means fart, and this led to the Latin word *pedere* meaning the verb to fart, and *peditum* the noun fart. The Indo-European *perd* led to the Greek word for fart πέρδομαι *perdomai*. It is also cognate with Sanskrit *pardate*, Avestan *parəδaiti*, Italian *fare un peto*, French "péter", Russian пердеть (perdet') and Polish "pierd".

The related Greek word *perdix* referred to a type of bird that made an explosive fart like sound when it was flushed from the brush when startled. While being incorporated from Greek to Old French it became *perdriz*, then Middle English *partrich*, and finally Modern English *partridge*. The final step would be to complete the circuitous history and modify it to the name *fartridge*!

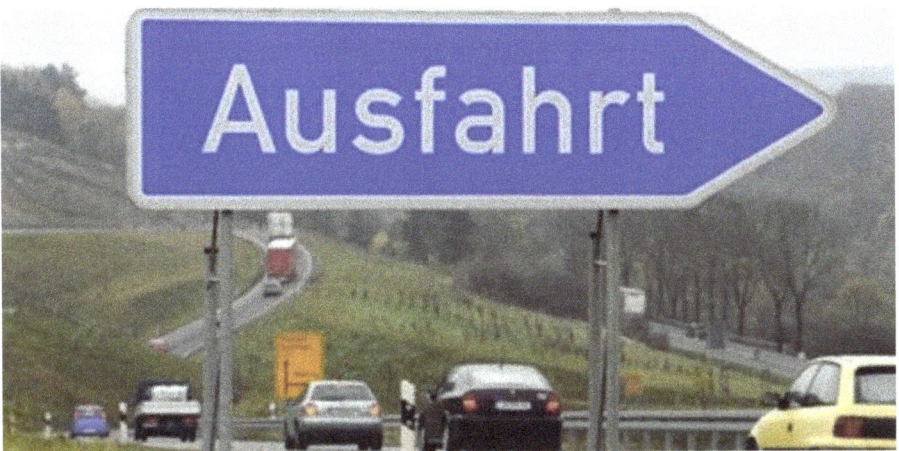

Traffic sign in Germany, Public Domain

The word fart is also found in other languages, but there it often has a different and unrelated meaning. In the Scandinavian languages it usually denotes speed or motion. In Danish and Norwegian it is often used in combination with other words that obscures the meaning even more. For example in Danish a *fartcertifikate* means a trade certificate.

In Norwegian a *fart plan* means a schedule. The Norwegian phrase *stå på fartin* pronounced as stop-a-fartin means ready to leave. Likewise the phrase *farts måler* pronounced as fart smeller refers to a speedometer. In Swedish a speed bump is called a *farthinder*. *Fartlek* is speed training by running at alternate intervals of fast and slow paces.

Likewise if you travel on a Scandinavian marine vessel you may see the control of engine speed labeled as *half fart* and *full fart* for half speed and full speed respectively. Fart kontrol zones are speed zones. In Germany a similar word *fahrt* means a journey, trip, tour, or passage. It is often seen in signs that say *einfahrt* (sounds like in-fart) and *ausfahrt* (sounds like out-fart) denoting entrance and exit respectively.

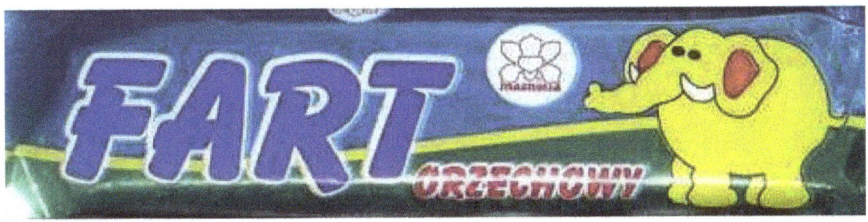

Artsy Fartsy: Cultural History of the Fart Volume One

In Spanish and Portuguese *fart* means an excess of anything, especially a food. One of the richest deserts they offer is called a *farte*, which means a fruit tarte in Spain and usually a sugar almond or cream cake in Portugal. In Italy the word *farto* means mattress. In Hungarian *fartaj* means buttocks. In Poland if you want to buy a popular candy bar with a name that means lucky you will be looking for a *Fart* bar.

Several languages have a number of different words for variations of a theme for which there is only one word in English. The word snow is one example where we have a singular word, but the Inuit, Eskimo, Aleut, Sami and other languages of the native people of the Arctic and northern latitudes may have hundreds of words.

When it comes to the word fart, the English language is very limited with just the singular word. I will not leap to the conclusion that the language that has the most words for fart needed to do so for necessity. Their population may or may not have the world's highest rate of fart production, but they certainly have the most descriptive fart words.

The Russian words for fart include *perdyozh* (first act of breaking wind), *perdun* (perpetrator and outcome), *perdil'nik* (place from where it comes), *Perun* (ancient God of wind), *bzdun* (silent fart), *bzdyukha* (silent fart as well as a stupid jerk). Some of the Russian verbs for the action of farting are particularly colorful. *Perdet'* (to fart with or without sound), *bzdet'* (to fart silently), *pereperdet* (to fart repeatedly), and my favorite word *nabzdet'sya* (to fart silently to one's complete and utter satisfaction!).

V. Physiology – Digestion and the Fart

Farts are ubiquitous, all living creatures generate gas from the cellular respiration of metabolism, and humans are no exception. The bacteria in your colonic flora generate microscopic nanofarts and microfarts, which collect into larger bubbles of gas in the bowel. They are intermixed with the atmospheric air swallowed throughout the day and particularly at meals.

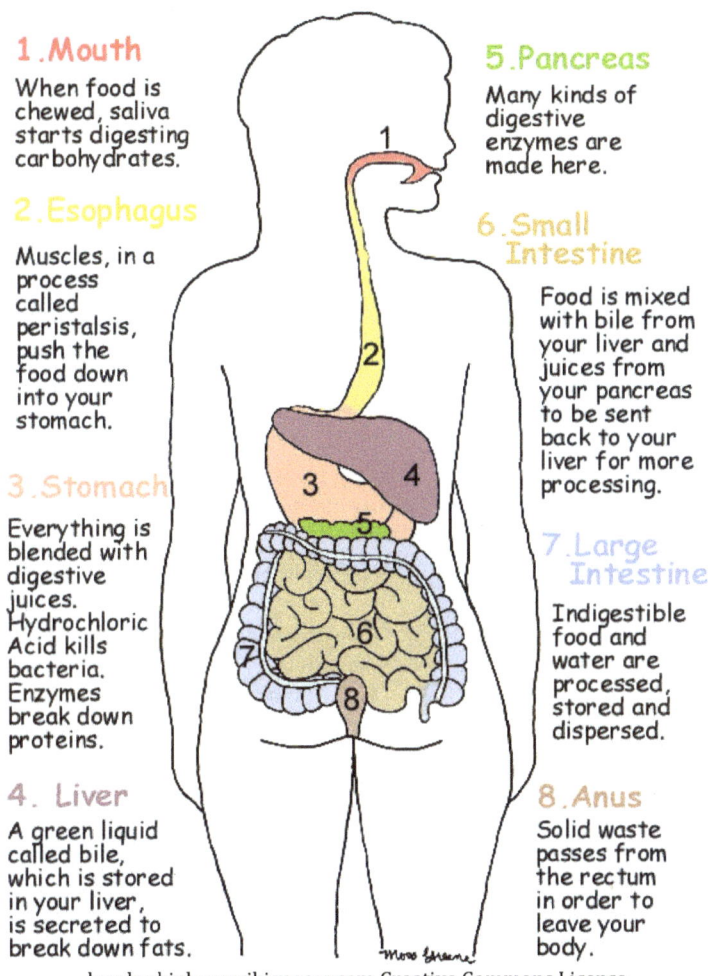

1. Mouth
When food is chewed, saliva starts digesting carbohydrates.

2. Esophagus
Muscles, in a process called peristalsis, push the food down into your stomach.

3. Stomach
Everything is blended with digestive juices. Hydrochloric Acid kills bacteria. Enzymes break down proteins.

4. Liver
A green liquid called bile, which is stored in your liver, is secreted to break down fats.

5. Pancreas
Many kinds of digestive enzymes are made here.

6. Small Intestine
Food is mixed with bile from your liver and juices from your pancreas to be sent back to your liver for more processing.

7. Large Intestine
Indigestible food and water are processed, stored and dispersed.

8. Anus
Solid waste passes from the rectum in order to leave your body.

hawkesbiology.wikispaces.com Creative Commons License

Aerophagia is universal and we swallow on average three to five milliliters (one teaspoonful) of air with every swallow. Even when we are not eating or drinking we regularly swallow the saliva we produce. The average human swallows over two thousand times a day. Chewing gum, hard candies, and use of chewing or smoking tobacco or other recreational products increase the volume of air swallowed. Drinking through a straw, directly from a can or bottle, or talking while eating, will also increase the amount of air swallowed. Ill-fitting dentures may also contribute to aerophagia. Another common source of swallowed air is contained within the foods we eat. An apple is forty percent air by volume, and bread is over sixty percent air by volume. If you compress an apple or a loaf of bread you will see that they a sizeable portion of their total volume is air. Whipped foods, soufflés, and baked goods, all have high air content.

Have you ever forgotten to put an ice cream container back in the freezer. Ice cream is typically forty percent air by volume and when it melts the air escapes and the full container is no longer full. By the way, the ice cream industry knows that adding air, known in the as overage, enhances the mouth feel texture of the ice cream and adds forty percent to the profit margin because ice cream is sold by volume, not by weight. Besides the swallowed air, additional gasses are produced during the enzymatic digestive processes, as well as the neutralization of gastric hydrochloric acid and pancreatic and duodenal bicarbonate. The end result is that a large volume of gasses transit the bowel and may be eliminated as a fart. Fortunately the vast majority of the gasses produced are absorbed by the gut and then into the bloodstream through diffusion into a solution. The gasses leave the bloodstream when they arrive at the alveoli of the lungs where they are exhaled. The chemical component gasses have very different properties of diffusion through the bowel wall and into the bloodstream.

Carbon dioxide readily diffuses and enters solution and is readily exhaled. It is the largest component of the volume of gas generated in the proximal intestinal tract. It is a major contributor to the temporary distention and discomfort that commonly occurs after a meal. Carbonation is also utilized as a common beverage enhancer and adds to the volume of carbon dioxide gas in the stomach. Carbon dioxide is the most rapidly absorbed component of intestinal gas and is the easiest to eliminate by simply exhaling it in the breath. As very little remains in the bowel, it is only a minor component of a fart.

The volume of gasses in the gastrointestinal tract is dependent on many factors. This includes the quantity and nature of foods ingested and the body's ability to synthesize and utilize specific enzymes for the various food types. The nature and quantity of the bacteria in the gut flora influences the nature of intestinal gas both by their own active metabolism and by their ability to aid or hinder the digestive enzymes and processes.

One of the most common causes of excess gaseousness is deficiency of the enzyme lactase. Lactase hydrolyses the complex disaccharide dairy sugar lactose into the readily absorbable monosaccharide sugars glucose and galactose. With insufficient lactase the sugar molecule is not metabolized by the digestive system but is instead metabolized by the gut flora, also known as the microbiome. This results in gas production, and may also give rise to cramps and diarrhea.

Artsy Fartsy: Cultural History of the Fart Volume One

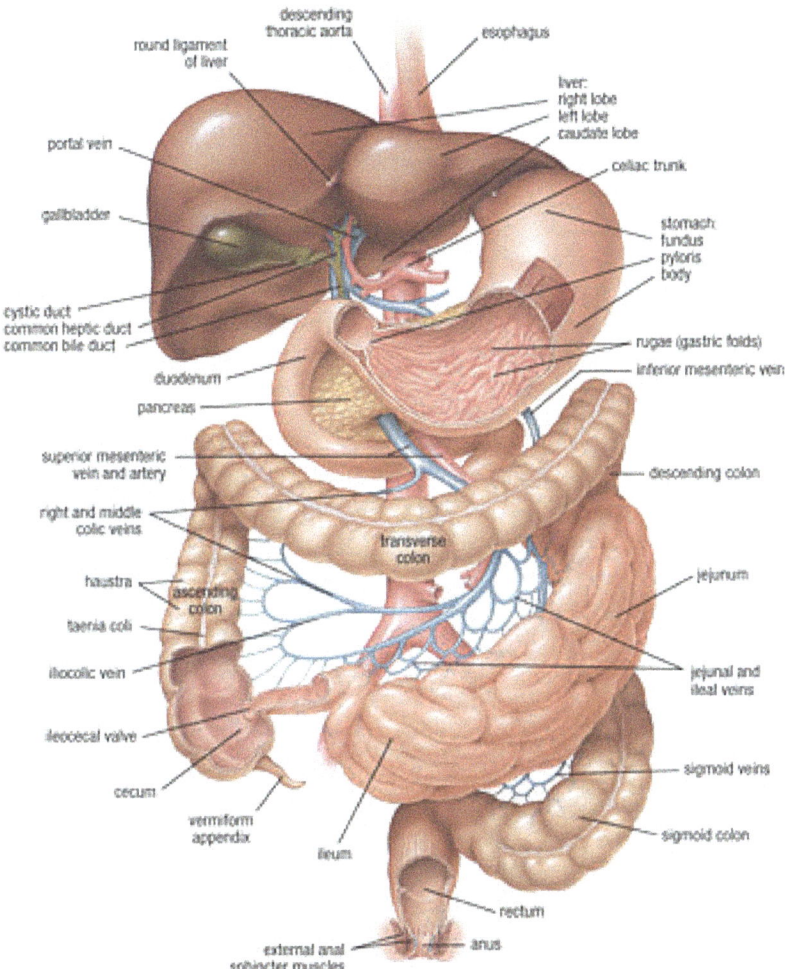

Openstax College courses.candelalearning.com Creative Commons License

Another food sugar that can cause excess gaseousness is commonly seen in fruit and is thus known as fructose. The human digestive system can handle a limited quantity of fructose at a time, and if the fruit intake exceeds this capacity the gut flora ferment this sugar with the release of gas, and often cramps and diarrhea.

That the microbes within our digestive tracts ferment foods that we have not fully digested is actually to our advantage, which is why the microbiome is considered essential to our good health. We can absorb some of the nutrients the microbes release in the fermentation process, including vitamins and bioactive molecules. We even use microbe fermentation in the preparation of many foods. When you add yeast to flour and watch the dough rise you are seeing the release of gasses from the fermentation process. The spongy character of bread and cakes, and why they are sixty percent air, is the result of gas production of the yeast fungus. The characteristic holes in Swiss cheese are the result of microbial gas production.

Artsy Fartsy: Cultural History of the Fart Volume One

The entire production of wines, beer, and other alcohol beverages are based on microbial fermentation. In a parallel universe, we are actually ingesting the waste product of microbial fermentation.

Before you believe that a delicious baked good dependent on yeast farts loses some of its culinary appeal, please read on. A French pastry delicacy known as Pets de Nonne, also called Pets de Sœurs, is accurately translated as Nun's farts. These delicacies are a dessert puff pastry dating from medieval times and made from butter, milk, flour, sugar, eggs and sometimes honey is added. They are traditionally pan fried in lard and then baked. Their lightness inspired their name in French, Pets de Nonne and Pets de Sœurs. Another baked good named for its association with the fart is Pumpernickel (German: Devil's Fart) bread. It is a heavy dark brown bread traditionally made with coarsely ground rye flour and whole rye berries. It has been long associated with the Westphalia region of Germany for over 500 years. Like most rye breads it is traditionally made with an acidic sourdough starter, which inhibits the rye amylase enzymes. The name is associated with the coarse bread giving rise to flatulence.

Beans are known as the musical fruit because of the gas they produce in all humans. The reason for this is that legumes contain complex sugars known as raffinose, verbascose, and stachyose. Humans and other animals lack the enzyme, called alpha galactosidase, needed to metabolize these complex sugars into absorbable simple sugars. Without the enzyme the complex sugars are fermented by the gut microbiome producing gas. Aplha galactosidase is now commercially available as a dietary enzyme supplement to reduce the gas production associated with specific foods such as legumes.

Another enzyme that humans do not posses is cellulase, without which we cannot digest the cellulose found in most plants and grasses. Herbivorous animals do have those enzymes, which is why they can subsist on grazing of grasses and forage. Ruminant animals also heavily rely on the metabolic activity of the gut flora. The large volumes of gasses formed in their multi-chambered stomach are believed to be more significant contributors to global warming than their flatulence. Another factor in gas production is the speed of gastrointestinal transit. Drugs, hormones, food products, and illness may influence this. The absorptive capacity and health of the mucosal lining, and the physical length of the individual's gastrointestinal tract also play a role. The often-quoted figure of twelve farts per day is a reasonable approximation of the average number of farts passed, but there is a very wide range of what is considered normal.

Besides the numerical quantity of farts passed per day is the question of what is considered a normal volume of gas passed. If you are familiar with physics, a series of natural laws were defined that express the relationship between temperature, pressure, and volume. The relationship between temperature and pressure is direct, i.e. the higher the temperature, the larger the volume of space a given number of molecules a gas would occupy. The expansion to a larger volume of occupied space may result in intestinal bloating, discomfort, and increased burping and farting. The relationship with pressure is indirect, i.e. the greater the pressure the smaller the volume.

We would rarely experience a change in intestinal gas volume based on temperature. On the contrary, we will often experience significant changes in volume due to pressure. Increases in pressure reduce the volume of gas, which is not a problem when it comes to the gut and our symptoms of gas. It can become a major problem when the pressure decreases and the gas volume increases. The atmospheric pressure changes rapidly as we go higher or lower from sea level. The effects on intestinal gas are seen in scuba divers, pilots, airplane passengers, mountain climbers, living at higher elevations, and even taking an elevator to the top of a skyscraper. When the pressure change is rapid, for example a scuba diver returning to the surface, or an astronaut on ascent to orbit, the consequences can be dramatic and life threatening and are known as barotrauma.

Most gasses that are commercially available (oxygen, helium, air, etc.) are compressed and contained in hardened metal canisters that can withstand very high pressure. This allows for significant savings of space, for example allowing scuba divers to have the equivalent of a roomful of air within a single tank. The intestinal tract is flexible and expandable to a degree, more like a balloon than a metal container. As such changes in the surrounding atmospheric pressure can result in large volume changes, which in the extreme of barotrauma may lead to perforation and rupture.

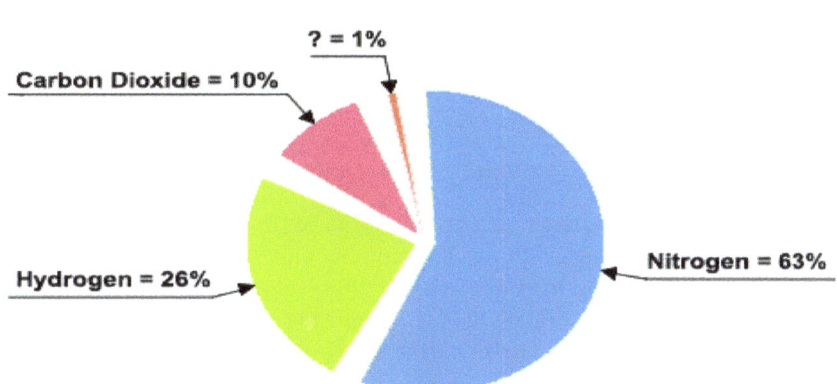

www.pyroenergen.com Creative Commons License

The fart would not be as notorious as it is if it were not for its aroma. Over ninety-nine percent of the gasses in a fart are odorless. While a number of individuals may have methane present in their farts, methane is odorless. If you smell a natural gas (methane) leak it is not the methane you smell, but an odorant gas added by the gas company as a safety precaution to give notice of danger.

Artsy Fartsy: Cultural History of the Fart Volume One

The majority of the aroma from a fart comes from hydrogen sulfide, skatole, indole, and aromatic fatty acids, the majority coming from the digestion of animal fats. While vegetarians may fart more than carnivores, the aroma is not nearly as pungent or offensive. For those interested in a more in-depth account of the fascinating natural history of intestinal gas (and its consequences of burping, bloating, and farting), the volume *To 'Air' is Human* is an enjoyable and definitive resource. In the meanwhile, before delving into the cultural history of the fart, a brief overview of digestion would be appropriate.

All of the attention on the physiologic origin of farts makes it sound like the primary purpose of the digestive tract is their creation for your annoyance or amusement. Of course, the purpose of the digestive tract is to support life by providing the nutrition and energy we need for all of our body functions. Intestinal gas is simply a natural waste product, and is rarely of consequence. As such, in my humble yet expert opinion, it should be utilized as a source of amusement or cultural enlightenment.

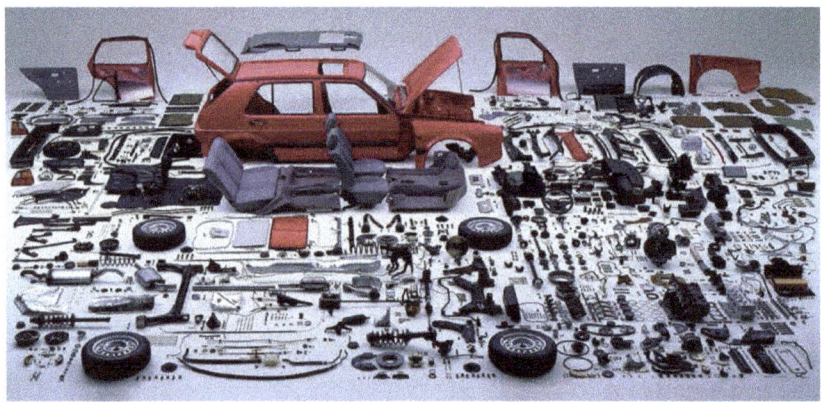

Creative Commons License

Perhaps the analogy is not the best one, but think of the digestive tract as the reverse of the assembly line, a disassembly line. A factory has a goal to be efficient and profitable, and may not win too many awards for architecture and beauty. So too with the digestive tract, the process has been refined over eons of evolution, yet still have its primitive origins and end products.

We begin our factory tour with a view much like you would get sitting in your car going through a car wash. Before you even go to the car wash, your brain has to make the conscious decision that this activity is what it wants to do. In the same manner, the brain begins the digestive process with the decision to satisfy its hunger call, or because an appetizing opportunity presents itself. When thinking about food and eating, the brain may activate the secretion of saliva and prime the digestive processes of the stomach and internal organs.

Artsy Fartsy: Cultural History of the Fart Volume One

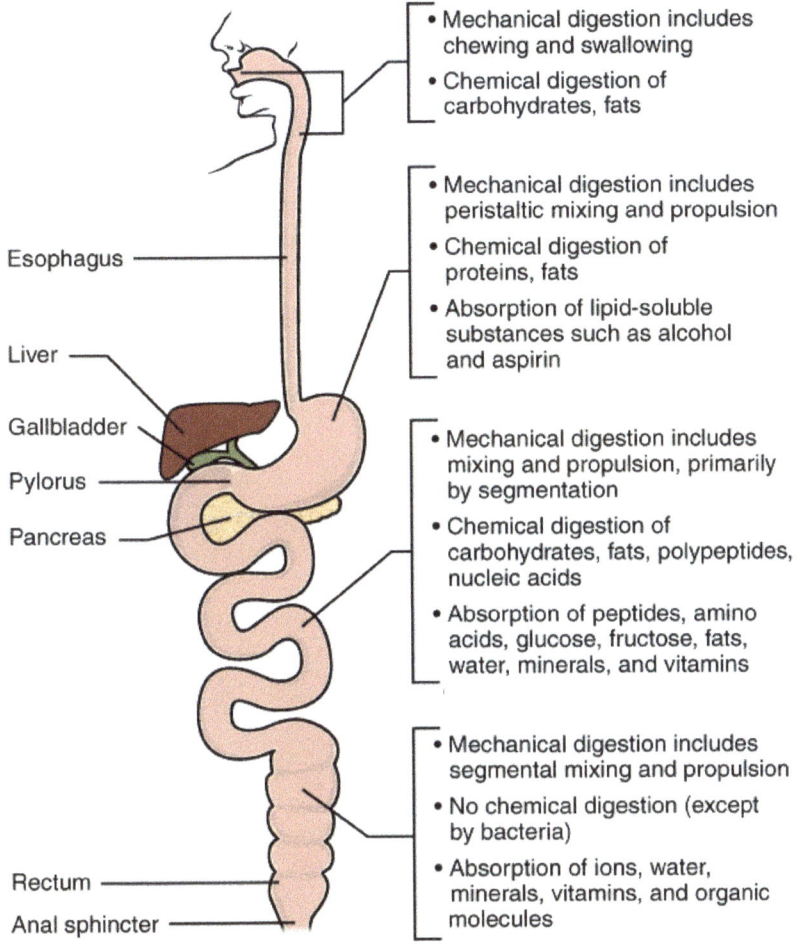

Openstax College courses.candelalearning.com Creative Commons License

Much like the water hoses and spray that greet your vehicle as you enter the beginning of the car wash tunnel, the entrance of food to the mouth receives a similar welcome. Jets of saliva are secreted from the ducts of the salivary glands located strategically around the oral cavity of the mouth. Saliva that is in the resting mouth is viscous and coats and protects the teeth and the inner surface of the mouth. The secreted saliva with eating or drinking is of a thinner more watery consistency. It has digestive enzymes including amylase to digest carbohydrates and lipase to digest fats.

If your carwash is as sophisticated as your digestive tract, it will have a crew to make sure your side mirrors are tucked in, and a prewash scrub of your tires and residue that would otherwise be difficult for the machinery to come. The teeth, jaws, and tongue work together in a remarkable and powerful dance with very few of the missteps which would be the dance equivalent of stepping on toes, the biting of the tongue.

The food has to be processed into smaller more manageable portions than that what is found on your plate. Your dining utensils of fork, knife, and spoon are just the preliminary, as the teeth do the real work in preparing food for the process of digestion. The teeth are subdivided into specific categories that have unique functions.

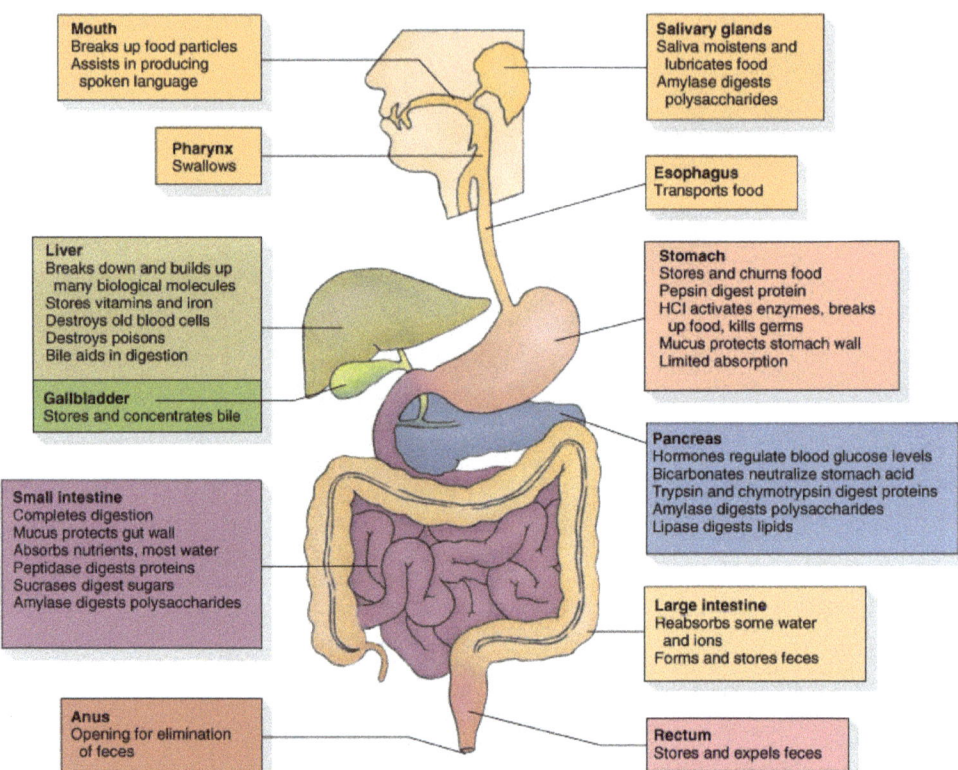

peptic-ulcer-disease-wikispaces.com Creative Commons License

The incisors cut the food as you bite into an apple, the canines tear the food apart as you dig into your pastrami sandwich, and your molars crush and grind the salad and crunchy vegetables you have as a side dish. The grinding and crushing break the plant cell walls apart that would otherwise protect its internal nutritious content from our digestive enzymes. They also increase the surface area of the food increasing their exposure to digestive acid and enzymes.

The chewing process assures that the saliva and its active enzymes are well mixed with the increased surface area of the food. They begin the process of breaking down the carbohydrates and lipids into their essential components to ready them for further digestion and absorption. The saliva also moistens the food and lubricates it for the coordinated swallowing motion of the tongue, teeth, palate and pharynx. These muscles and organs work together to roll it into an easy to swallow food bolus. The muscles of the swallowing process include those that protect the larynx and airway. By having the epiglottis close off the passageway to the trachea, bronchi, and lungs, it prevents aspiration into the airways as the food and saliva swallow takes place.

The coordinated action is developed with age, which is why small children should avoid foods, such as nuts, grapes, larger oval or rounded candies. These foods, if inappropriately swallowed into the airway, can lead to fatal choking episodes. Tragically a number of children die because the oval or rounded shape can completely block the airway. An irregular shaped object, which can be life threatening, rarely completely obstructs the airway and usually allows some air to pass.

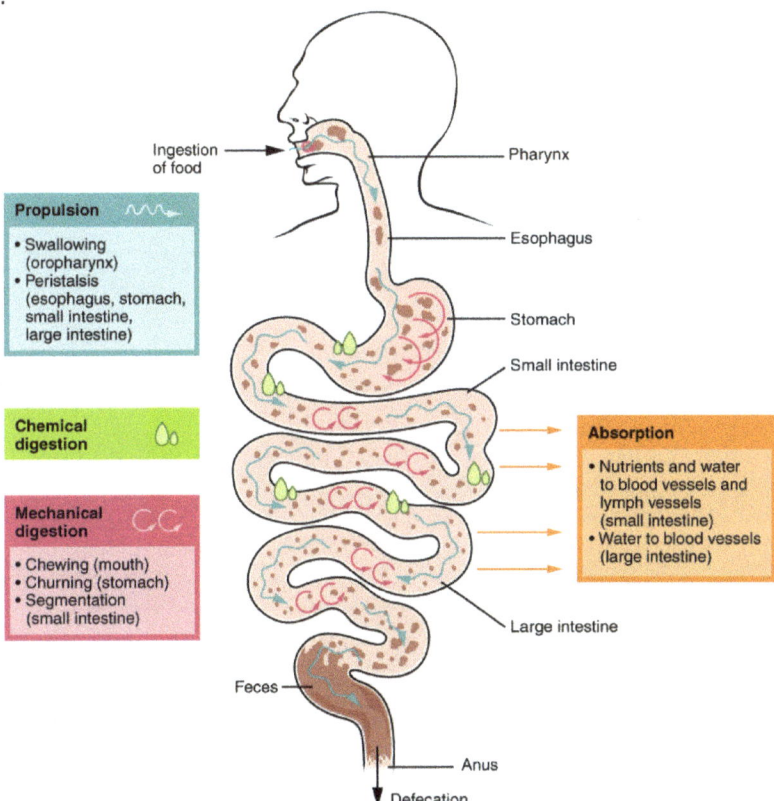

Openstax College philschatz.com Creative Commons License

The complicated swallowing neuromuscular coordination can also be affected by neurological disorders, stroke, surgery or other conditions, which may lead to the risk of aspiration. Once swallowed, the food bolus is propelled down the esophagus by coordinated snakelike muscular action, known as peristalsis. It is not recommended, but the swallowing mechanism is so effective that you can swallow against gravity while standing on your head.

The muscular valve at the junction of the esophagus and stomach is called the lower esophageal sphincter. The lower esophageal sphincter is designed to allow food and fluid to enter the stomach, with the door closed behind them once they leave the esophagus. If the valve opens at the wrong time, gastric acid, digestive enzymes, and food can flow back into the esophagus. This can lead to symptoms of heartburn or mucosal damage. If the refluxed material goes all the way into the airway hoarseness, sore throat, aspiration, choking, or pneumonia can develop. If it occurs frequently gastroesophageal reflux disease (GERD) can predispose to a change in the tissue lining the esophagus. The growth of intestinal type tissue is called a Barrett esophagus, and is at a higher risk of cancer development than the normal lining tissue. Individuals with Barrett esophagus are treated for GERD and monitored closely for pre-malignant changes.

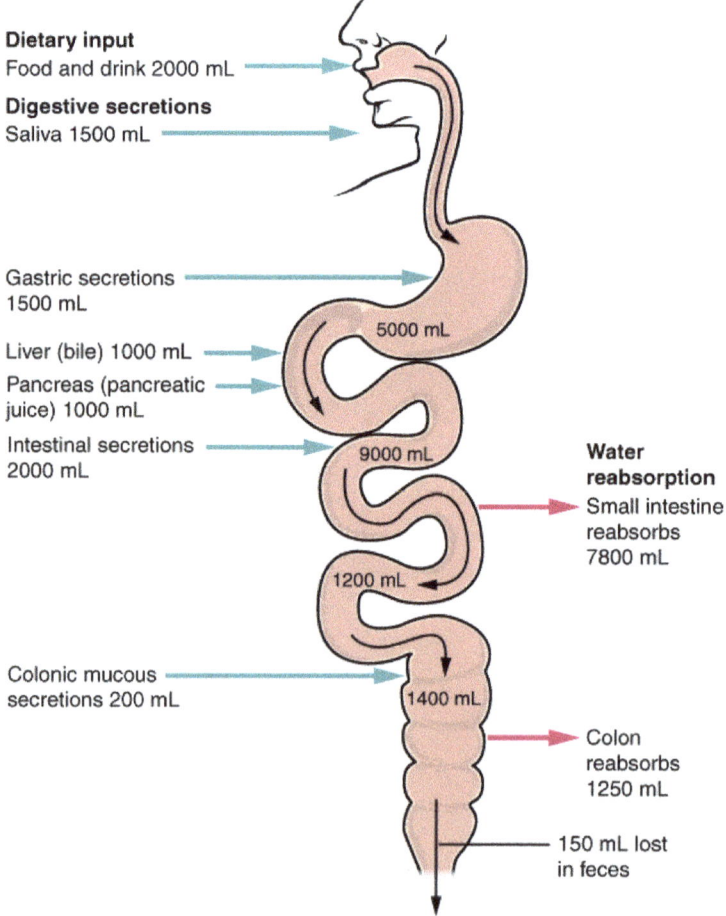

Openstax College courses.candelalearning.com Creative Commons License

The stomach is a churning cauldron of muscular mixing contractions, concentrated acid secretion, and potent digestive enzymes. The Vagus nerve and gut hormones play a key role in the intricate balance of enzymes, acid, nutrients, and motility. When the conditions are right, the pyloric sphincter of the stomach opens to allow the acid, enzyme, and food mixture to exit. This digestive material is now called chyme as it enters the first portion of the small intestine, known as the duodenum. In Greek, this means the width equivalent to twelve fingers, which is what its small size would measure using your digits. For its small size, the duodenum plays an amazing and complex part.

The highly acidic chyme would quickly damage the lining of the duodenum if it did not respond quickly with the pouring on, much like a fire extinguisher, of sodium bicarbonate. The sodium bicarbonate is produced in the duodenum itself, as well as the pancreas. The sodium bicarbonate produced in the pancreas is released through the pancreatic duct, which empties into the duodenum through the Ampulla of Vater.

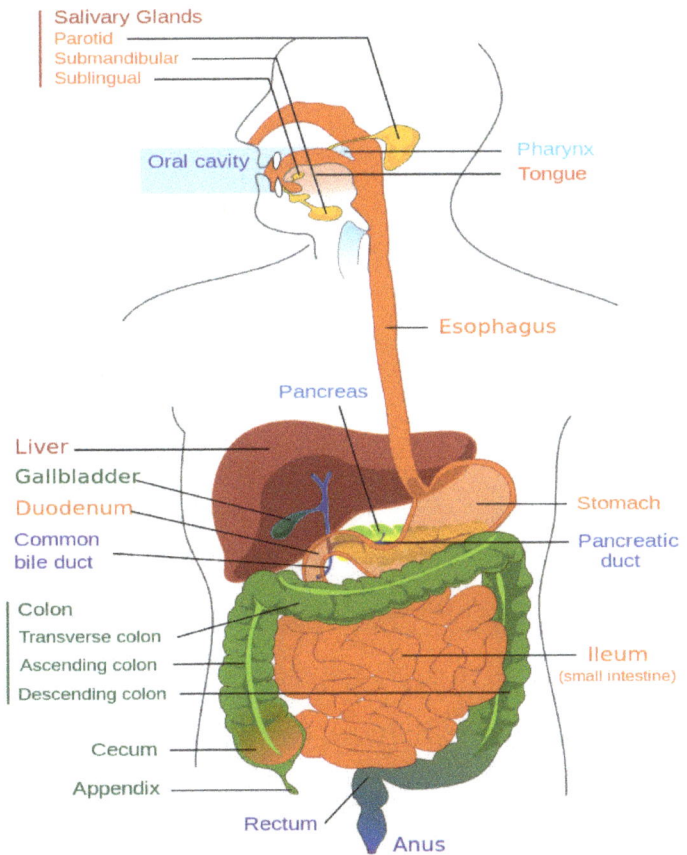

Mariana Ruiz LadyofHats, edited by Joaquim Alves Gaspar Creative Commons License

The fire extinguisher analogy shares another aspect of the story. Perhaps you made a fire extinguisher in a science class, or home experiment, by adding baking soda that contains sodium bicarbonate and vinegar that contains acetic acid. This is the same type of reaction that takes place in the duodenum, when the hydrochloric acid of the stomach meets the sodium bicarbonate released to neutralize it. When the two react they produce water, sodium chloride (salt), and large quantities of carbon dioxide. The carbon dioxide is released as large volumes of gas that appears as a bubbles arising from the reaction. The carbon dioxide is used as a fire extinguisher in the science experiment since it is heavier than air, and cuts off the oxygen supply that the fire requires. In the human duodenum, the carbon dioxide generated as a side product of acid neutralization only serves to bloat and distend the gut with gas. The body is pretty remarkable in getting rid of the bloat fairly quickly, in that it absorbs the carbon dioxide into the bloodstream where it travels to the lungs to be exhaled.

Major Digestive Enzymes

Enzyme	Produced In	Site of Release	pH Level
Carbohydrate Digestion:			
Salivary amylase	Salivary Glands	Mouth	Neutral
Pancreatic amylase	Pancreas	Small Intestine	Basic
Maltase	Small intestine	Small intestine	Basic
Protien Digestion:			
Pepsin	Gastric glands	Stomach	Acidic
Trypsin	Pancreas	Small intestine	Basic
Peptidases	Small Intestine	Small intestine	Basic
Nucleic Acid Digestion:			
Nuclease	Pancreas	Small intestine	Basic
Nucleosidases	Pancreas	Small intestine	Basic
Fat Digestion:			
Lipase	Pancreas	Small intestine	Basic

commons.wikimedia.org Creative Commons License

The bile ducts from the liver join the duct from the pancreas bringing digestive enzymes and bicarbonate that enter the duodenum through the Ampulla of Vater. Within the ampulla lies the muscular sphincter of Oddi. The name sounds like a character from the story of the Wizard of Oz, and that would be an appropriate analogy. The coordinated release of hormones, enzymes, motility and vagal input is nothing short of wizardry. Subconsciously, your body can sense exactly what nutrients you have ingested. It responds by releasing the best recipe of enzymes, acid in the stomach, and bicarbonate in the duodenum, adjusting the pH as necessary. It adds just the right amount of bile to the mix, controls the timing and volume of stomach emptying, and controls the speed of transit and intensity of mixing contractions through the length of the intestinal tract. The majority of the sensing and control feedback takes place in a small confined space the width of twelve fingers, the duodenum.

The breakdown products of the digestive process are absorbed through a sea of finger like projections called the villi. It looks like a field of waving wheat stalks, each upstanding villus is ready to use its enzymes and absorptive capacity to absorb nutrients. If you looked under the microscope you would find that each villus has thousands of even smaller villi on its surface, given the appropriate name of microvilli. All of these folds of absorptive tissue, if flattened out, would provide the equivalent absorptive capacity of a championship tennis court. A quote from Mark Twain also illustrates the concept of surface area: "If Switzerland were ironed flat it would be a very large country". The long intestinal tunnel of eagerly awaiting absorptive villi is about twenty feet long, and it is an amazingly efficient system of digestion and absorption.

If injured, the ability of the small bowel to digest and absorb nutrients is compromised. A condition that temporarily damages the small intestine, such as a viral or bacterial gastroenteritis often called stomach flu, can cause a blunting or shortening of the villi. The villous blunting will also lead to the loss of digestive enzymes that reside on the villi. Without the ability to digest and absorb nutrients, the unabsorbed material can cause what is known as an osmotic diarrhea. This is one of the reasons people are often advised to avoid dairy products for a week or so after stomach flu to allow the villi and enzymes to recover. If you eat or drink lactose without waiting until the recovery is complete, you may end up with symptoms of temporary lactose intolerance such as gas and diarrhea.

When the liquid chyme leaves the jejunum and ileum of the small intestine, it goes through the ileocecal valve to enter the colon. In the cecum of the colon lies the infamous appendix, which for thousands of years mystified science as to its purpose. It looks like its function has finally, and only very recently, been identified. It stores a reservoir of intestinal bacteria, representing the healthy gut microbiome, from which the gut flora can be replenished after a bout of intestinal dysentery.

The gut microbiome is much more important than most people give it credit for. The microbes of the body far outnumber the number of human cells. In fact, if you simply go by the number of cells and not their mass, they outnumber human cells by ten to one. In other words, you as a living system are only ten percent human, and ninety percent microbes! The vast majority of the microbes living within and on us are commensals. This means that they are engaged with us in a symbiotic relationship from which we both benefit. They are able to process foods that would otherwise be indigestible, and convert them to absorbable nutrients and metabolites. It is not an understatement to say that they are a requirement for our health and wellbeing. The gut microbiome also plays a very important role in the gut-brain-microbiome-axis, which provides for the communication of important information between the three. Many experts now include food as the fourth component of this important communication axis.

The colon, unlike the small intestine, is less involved in the digestion of foods and nutrients. It is primarily involved in the absorption of water and sodium, as well as some fat-soluble vitamins such as vitamin K. The colon removes the excess moisture from the watery chyme, and the stool solidifies as it transits the gut. The ability to conserve water is very important, and without this ability the risk of dehydration would be substantially increased. The fecal material of the stool is stored in the rectum and sigmoid colon awaiting the right opportunity to be eliminated through defecation.

A process or illness that impairs the colon's absorption of water will lead to more fluid in the stool and diarrhea. The loss of water and electrolytes as a consequence of diarrhea unfortunately remains a life threatening condition in many parts of the world, especially for infants and children. If the elimination of the feces is delayed, the moisture continues to be absorbed and the stools can become harder resulting in constipation. Constipation itself can be self-perpetuating as it aggravates the situation because the stools become harder and more difficult to pass the longer they remain in the colon. The more common treatments for constipation attempt to increase the moisture content of the stool.

The feces excreted can provide information about bowel health. For most people going about their daily activities, the passage of the feces itself is the end of the story of digestion. The human digestive system, like that of other animals, does not remove all of the available nutrients from food. For other organisms, including the common housefly, the feces are thus an available source of nutrition. For them the elimination of feces is just the beginning of their story of digestion, and can play an important role in the transmission of disease back to humans.

VI. Chronology of Fart in the Arts

Hieronymus Bosch

Hieronymus Bosch (c. 1450 – 1516) was a Dutch artist known for his use of colorful imagery to illustrate religious concepts. His most famous triptych is *The Garden of Earthly Delights*. It illustrates a scene depicting paradise with Adam and Eve on the left panel, numerous nude figures, fruit and birds depicting the earthly delights on the middle panel, and hell with depictions of the punishments of sinners on the right panel. In the central panel a nude figure is farting roses, and in the right panel of hell a nude male is playing the flute from his rear end.

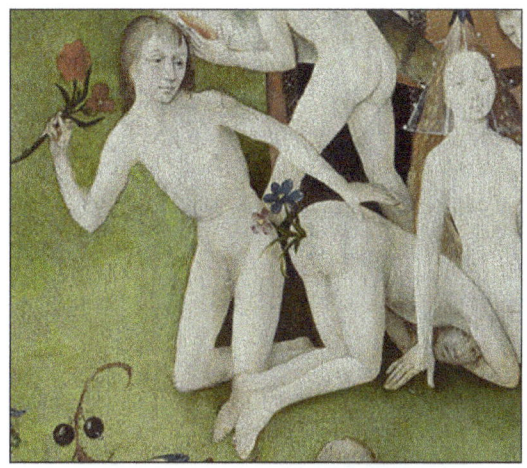

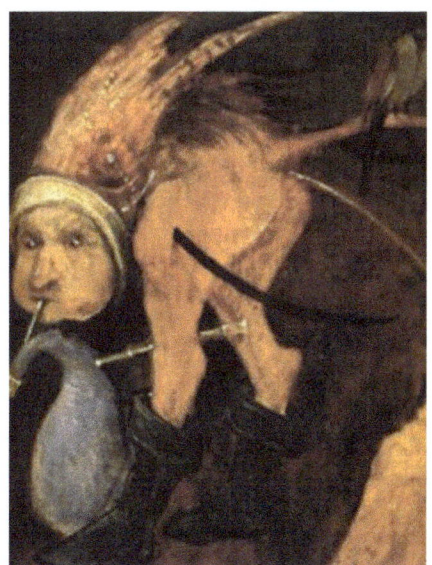

The Garden of Earthly Delights. Hieronymus Bosch between 1480 and 1505, Museo del Prado, Madrid
Public Domain

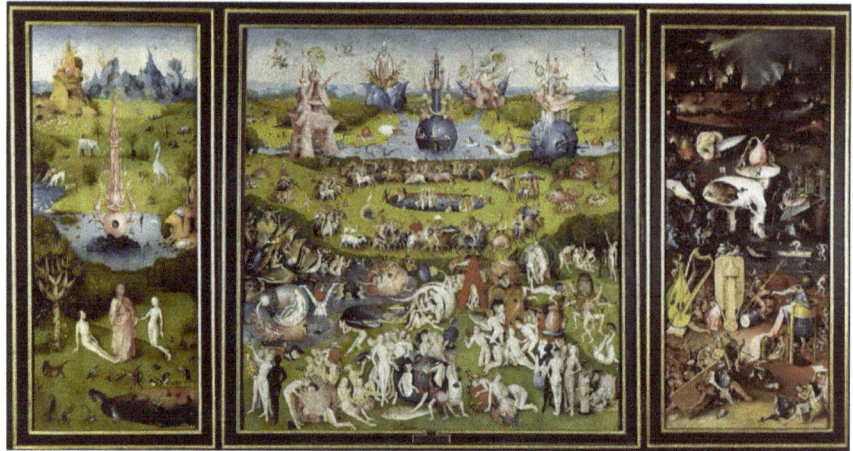

The Garden of Earthly Delights. Hieronymus Bosch between 1480 and 1505, Museo del Prado, Madrid
Public Domain

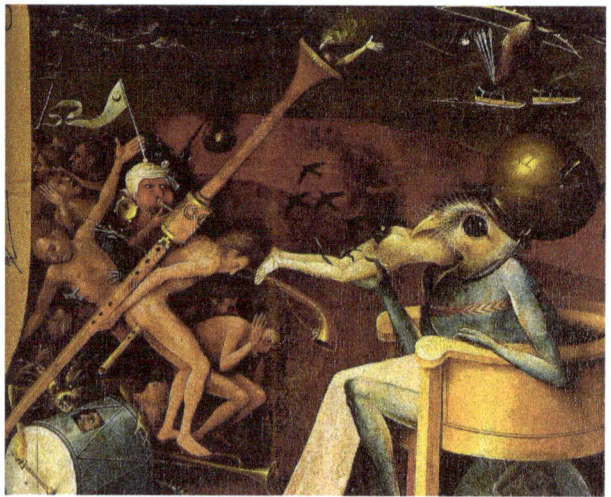

Famous Quotation:

"And what is the potential man, after all? Is he not the sum of all that is human? Divine, in other words?"

Michelangelo di Lodovico Buonarroti Simoni

Michelangelo di Lodovico Buonarroti Simoni (1475 - 1564) was a leading Italian Renaissance sculptor, painter, engineer, architect, and poet. The *Creation of Adam* is considered his masterpiece and was painted on the ceiling of the Sistine Chapel at the Vatican in Rome. The painting illustrates the biblical passage where God breathes life into Adam, or transmits the spark of life through his finger.

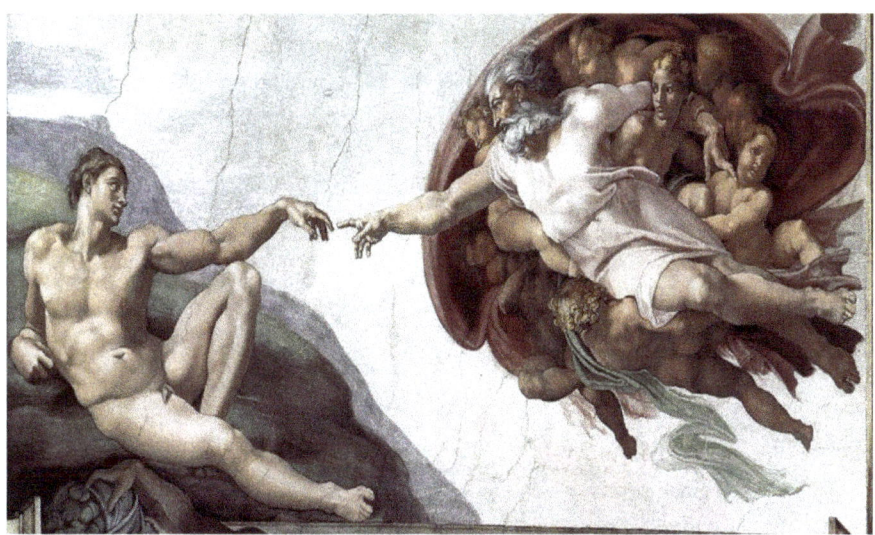
Michelangelo Buonarroti c. 1511 Sistine Chapel Public Domain

There really isn't a factual fart behind this masterpiece of incredible artistic talent. Poetic license to include it is taken because many parodies of this masterpiece by Michelangelo appear to have God beckoning to Adam, and the viewer, to pull his finger.

Famous Quotations:

"If people knew how hard I had to work to gain my mastery, it would not seem so wonderful at all."
"If you knew how much work went into it, you wouldn't call it genius. "
"The greater danger for most of us lies not in setting our aim too high and falling short; but in setting our aim too low, and achieving our mark."
"I saw the angel in the marble and carved until I set him free."
"Every block of stone has a statue inside it and it is the task of the sculptor to discover it"
"I am still learning."
"The sculpture is already complete within the marble block, before I start my work. It is already there, I just have to chisel away the superfluous material."
"Genius is eternal patience"

Pieter Bruegel (Brueghel) the Elder

Pieter Bruegel (Brueghel) the Elder (c. 1525 –1569) was an artist of the Flemish Renaissance known for his peasant scenes and painted religious works. Using artistic humor he created some of the early images dealing with the sensitive subject of social protest in art history. The painting *Netherlandish Proverbs* illustrates a number of Dutch proverbs and sayings.

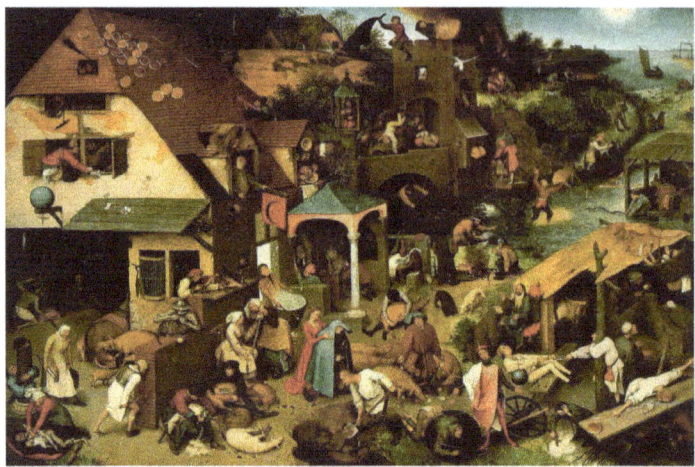

Netherlandish Proverbs illustrates over 112 Dutch proverbs. 1559 Pieter Bruegel (Brueghel) the Elder Staatliche Museen, Berlin Public Domain

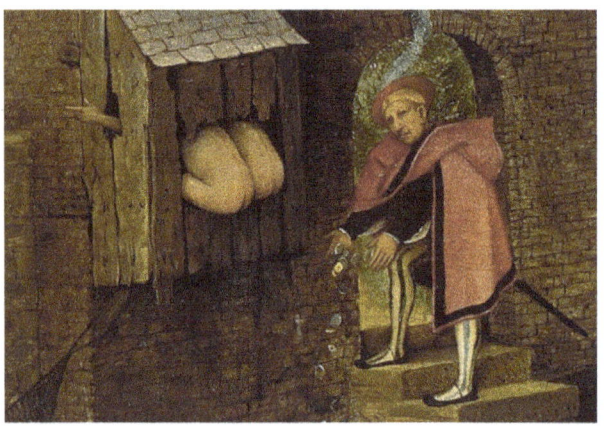

The proverb "It hangs like a privy over a ditch" has a meaning, which is self-evident and can be taken literally. On his deathbed Pieter Bruegel ordered his wife to burn his most powerful paintings of protest to protect his family from the persecutions raging from conflicts between the Protestant Reformation and the Catholic Church. The exposed buttocks above the river illustrate two proverbs. "They both crap and fart through the same hole" is a proverb that illustrates the meaning that the people discussed were in agreement.

Medieval Manuscripts

Medieval manuscripts were often texts of learned knowledge that needed to be transmitted to the next generation. They often exhibited illustrations of natural processes, surgical procedures, and anatomy that would not be considered works purely for art alone.

Artsy Fartsy: Cultural History of the Fart Volume One

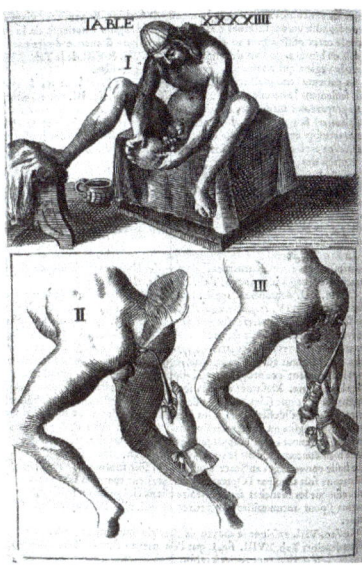

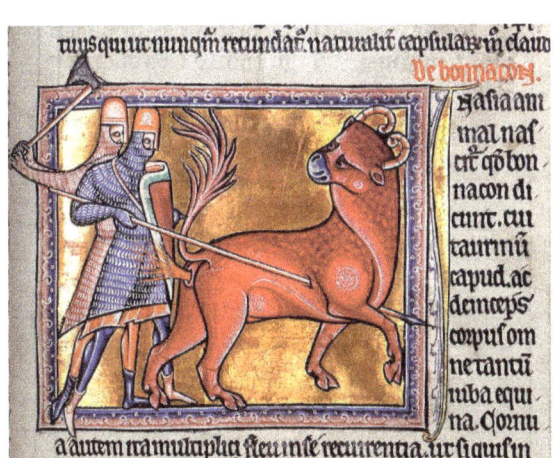

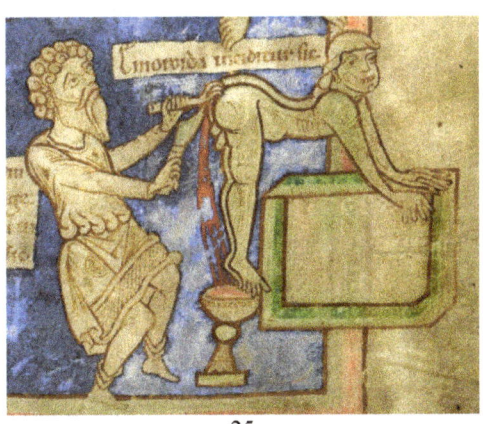

Artsy Fartsy: Cultural History of the Fart Volume One

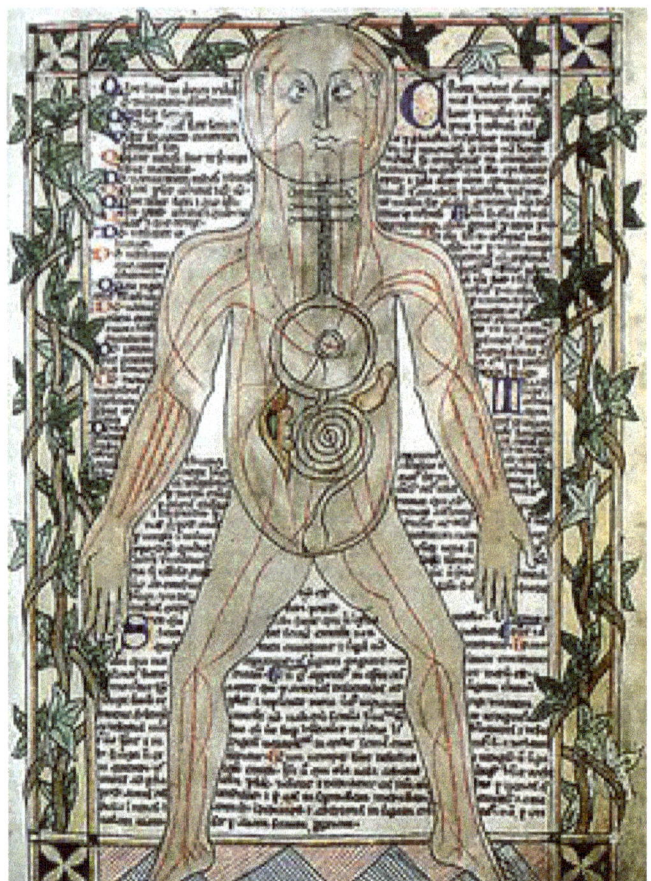

Francisco Goya

Francisco José de Goya y Lucientes, more commonly known as Francisco Goya (1746-1828) was a Spanish artist who has been considered as the last of the Old Masters and the first of the modernists. He created a set of prints entitled *Los Caprichos* in 1797-1798 that was a criticism of society. Goya's description of his work was that it depicted "the innumerable foibles and follies to be found in any civilized society, and from the common prejudices and deceitful practices which custom, ignorance or self-interest have made usual".

Ironically, Goya withdrew the prints from public sale and circulation, and only in his later life did he disclose that he did so because of intimidation from the Spanish Inquisition. The Tribunal of the Office of the Inquisition was established in 1478 but was not formally abolished until 1834.

Artsy Fartsy: Cultural History of the Fart Volume One

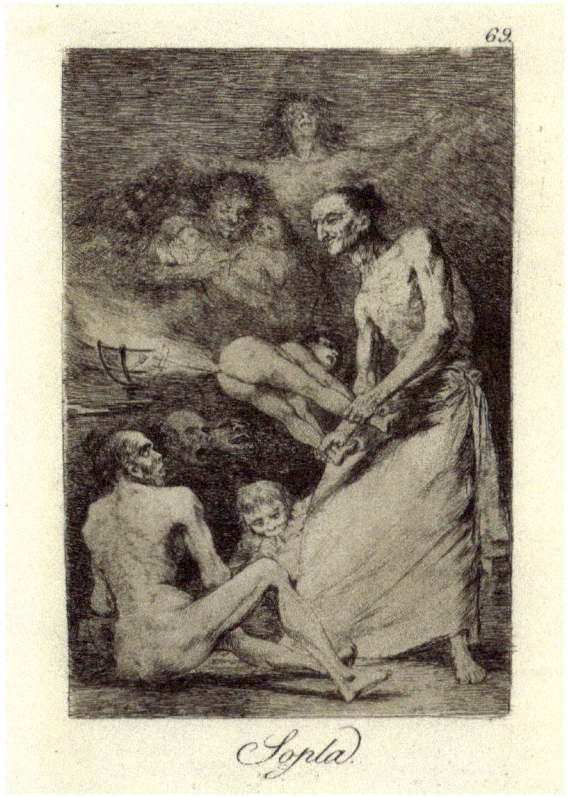
Goya -Sopla Gust the wind Capricho Public Domain

Wolfgang Amadeus Mozart

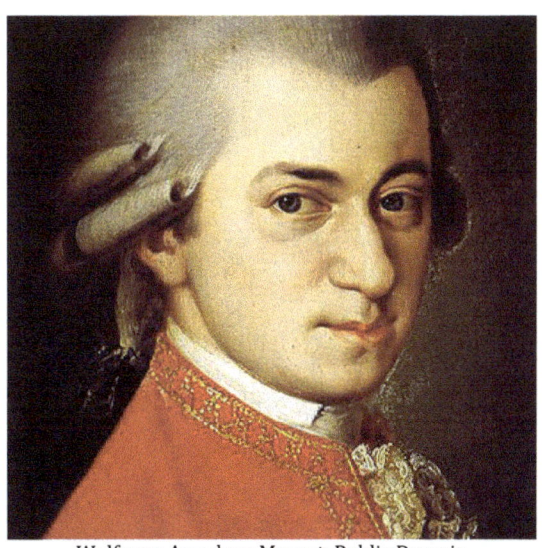
Wolfgang Amadeus Mozart, Public Domain

Wolfgang Amadeus Mozart (1756 – 1791) was a child prodigy who maintained a juvenile sense of humor throughout his relatively short but incredibly prolific and talented life. Some of his musical notes suggest the playing of a human wind instrument.

He was obsessed with jokes about farts, farting, feces, analingus, and copraphilia. His early death and paupers burial makes one wonder if his obsessions and jocular fantasy contributed to his estrangement from others and his tragic downfall.

He wrote the following poem for his dear mother in a letter from 1778:
"Oh mother of mine:
Butter is fine.
Praise and thanks be to Him,
We're alive and full of vim.
Through the world we dash,
Though we're rather short of cash,
But we don't find this provoking
And none of us are choking.
Besides, to the people I'm tied
Who carry their muck inside
And let it out if they are able,
Both before and after the table.
At night of farts there is no lack,
Which let off, forsooth, with a powerful crack.
The king of farts came yesterday
Whose farts smelt sweeter than the may.
His voice, however, was no treat
And he himself was in a heat.
Well, now we've been over a week away
And we've been shitting everyday.
Wendling, no doubt, is in a rage
That I haven't composed a single page;
But when I cross the Rhine once more,
I'll surely dash home through the door
And, least he call me mean and petty,
I'll finish off his four quartetti.
The concerto for Paris I'll keep, tis' more fitting.
I'll scribble it there someday when I'm shitting.
Indeed I swear 'twould be far more fun
With the Webers around the world to run
Then go with those bores, you know whom I mean.
When I think of their faces, I get the spleen.
But I suppose it must be and off we shall toddle,
Though Weber's arse I prefer to Ramm's noodle.

A slice of Weber's arse is a thing
I'd rather have than Monsieur Wendling.
With our shitting God we cannot hurt,
And least of all if we bite the dirt.
We are honest birds, all of a feather,
We have summa summarum eight eyes together
Not counting those on which we sit.
But now I must rest a bit
From Rhyming. Yet this I must add,
That on Monday I'll have the honor, egad,
To embrace you and kiss your hands so fair.
But first in my pants I'll shit, I swear
Your faithful child, With distemper wild.
Trazom."

Famous Quotations:

"The music is not in the notes, but in the silence between."
"Neither a lofty degree of intelligence nor imagination nor both together go to the making of genius. Love, love, love, that is the soul of genius."
"Forgive me, Majesty. I am a vulgar man! But I assure you, my music is not."
"When I am ..... completely myself, entirely alone... or during the night when I cannot sleep, it is on such occasions that my ideas flow best and most abundantly. Whence and how these ideas come I know not nor can I force them."
"To talk well and eloquently is a very great art, but that an equally great one is to know the right moment to stop."
"It is a mistake to think that the practice of my art has become easy to me. I assure you, dear friend, no one has given so much care to the study of composition as I. There is scarcely a famous master in music whose works I have not frequently and diligently studied."
"A man of ordinary talent will always be ordinary, whether he travels or not; but a man of superior talent will go to pieces if he remains forever in the same place."
"I pay no attention whatever to anybody's praise or blame. I simply follow my own feelings."

James Gillray

James Gillray (1757-1815) was a noted English satirical cartoonist and printmaker. The illustration shows experiments with nitrous oxide (laughing gas) at the Royal Institution. The subject of the inhalation of nitrous oxide releases a blast of gas as a fart.

Humphrey Davy noted for his work on the chemistry of gasses is working the bellows. Etching is entitled "Scientific Researches!—New Discoveries in PNEUMATICKS!—or—an Experimental Lecture on the Powers of Air," published 1802.

Although laughing gas was an agent that inspired frivolity and merriment it eventually contributed to the development of anesthesia and a surgical revolution. Unfortunately it took many decades before anyone followed Humphrey Davy's suggestion that it be investigated as an anesthetic. The barbarity and fear of the excruciating pain of surgery in the day before anesthesia cannot be overemphasized. Other cartoons also showed his fascination with chemistry, and gasses in particular. He also illustrated the concern of bloating and distention with digestion and overeating.

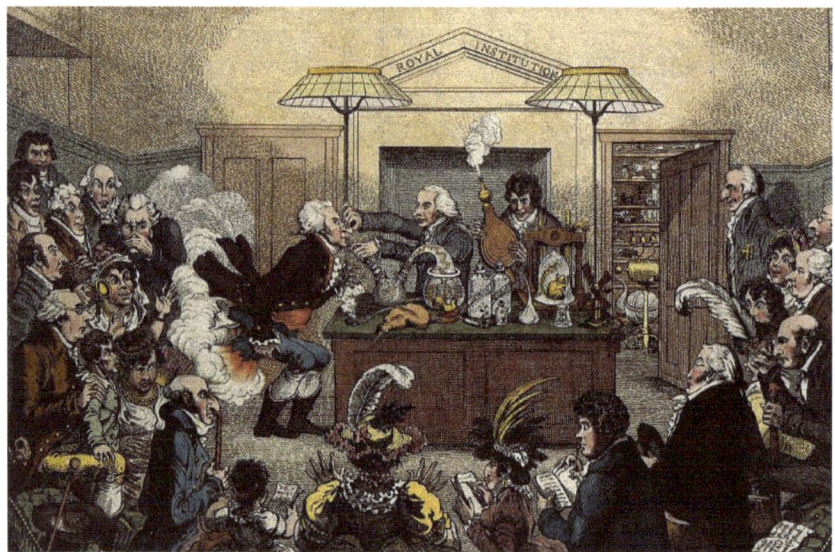

James Gillray, Public Domain

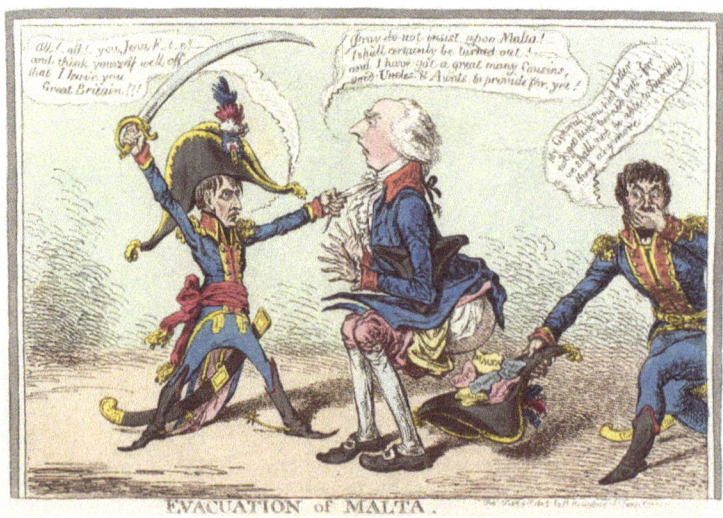

James Gillray, Evacuation of Malta

Artsy Fartsy: Cultural History of the Fart Volume One

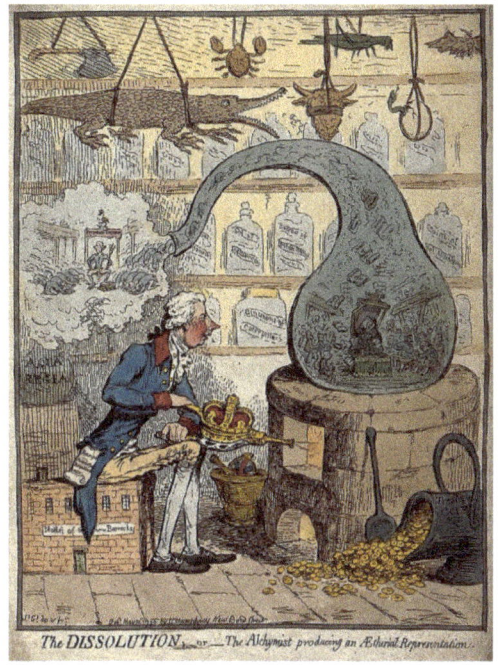

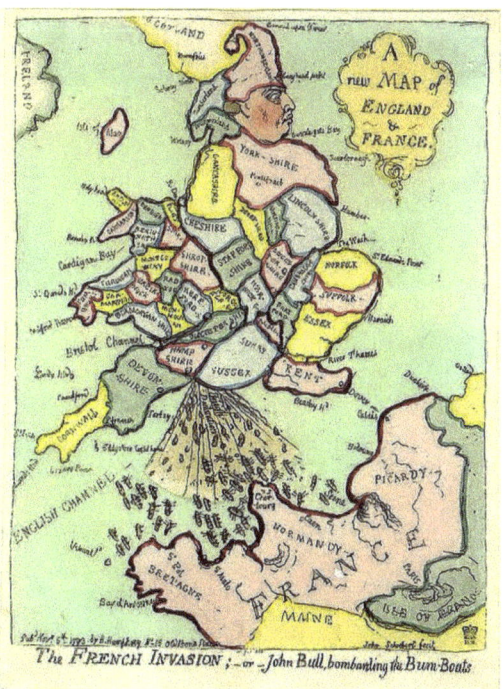

James Gillray, The French Invasion Public Domain

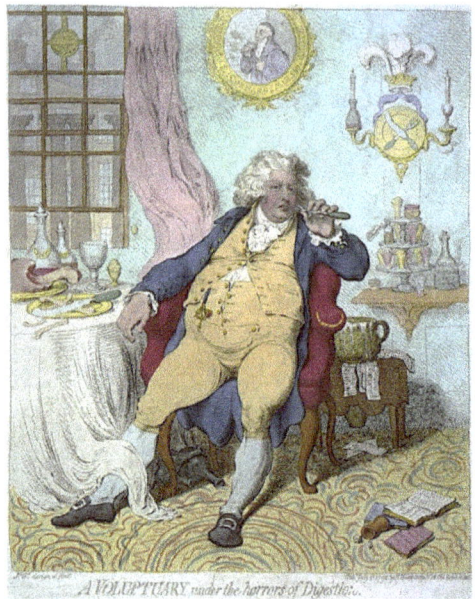
James Gillray, Public Domain

Gillray was not alone in his satirical cartoons. William Dent, Willam Wells, and others often took a scatological turn in their biting satire.

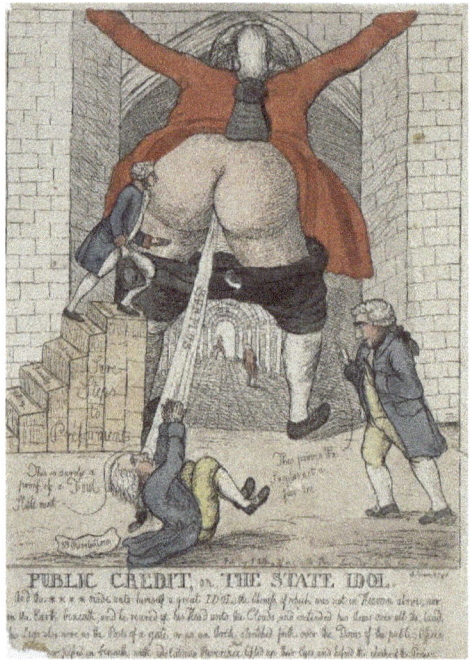
William Dent, Public Credit or the State Idol Public Domain

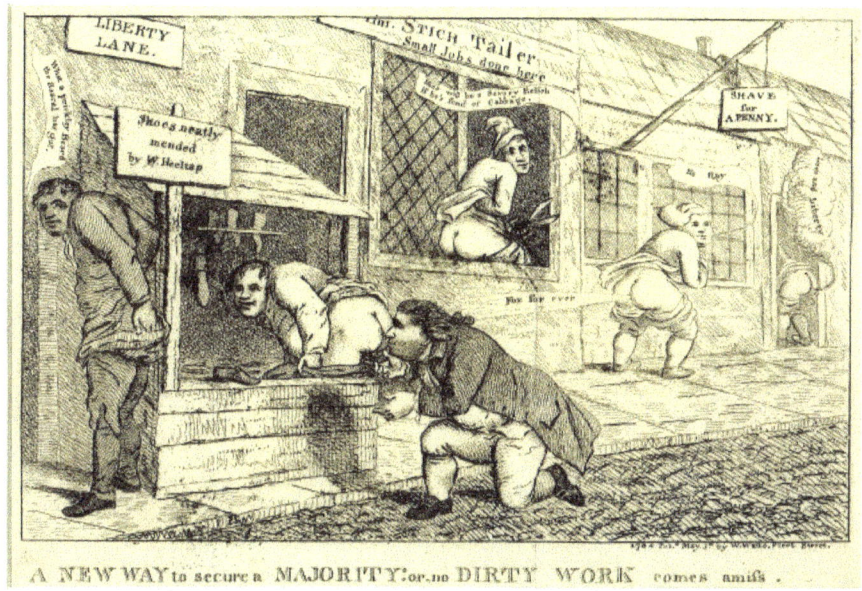
William, Wells, A New Way to Secure a Majority 1784 Public Domain

Louis-Léopold Boilly

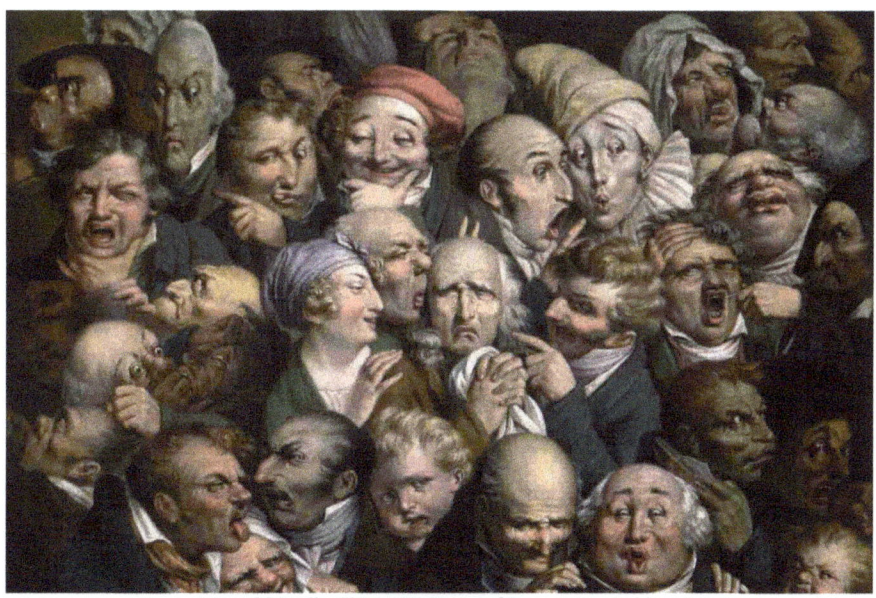
Louis-Léopold Boilly *Thirty-Six Faces of Expression*. Public Domain

Louis-Léopold Boilly (1761–1845) was a French painter, draftsman, and popular portrait painter who vividly documented French middle-class social life. His life and times spanned some of the most dramatic moments of French history including the French monarchs, the French Revolution, the Age of Napoleon, the Bourbon Restoration and the July Monarchy.

He was a very popular and celebrated figure in his time. In spite of his popularity, at the peak of the revolutionary Terror in 1794 his life was in danger. Boilly was tried and condemned by the Committee of Public Safety for the erotic nature of his work. He was spared punishment by the discovery in his home of additional works of art including the more patriotic *Triumph of Marat* (Musée des Beaux Arts, Lille).

Richard Newton

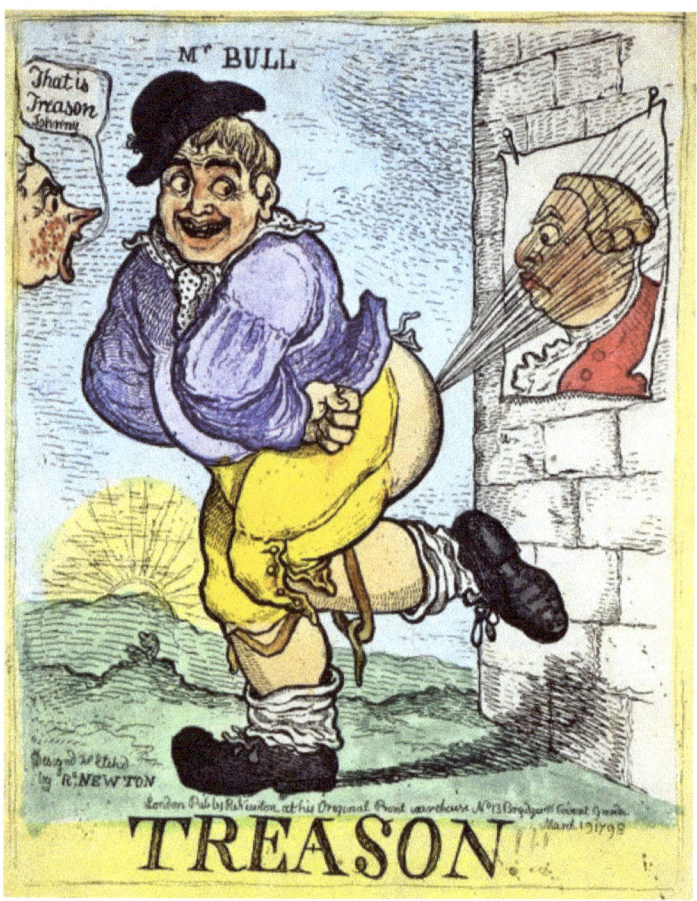

Richard Newton, Public Domain

Richard Newton (1777-1798 was a brilliant British cartoonist and political satirist who died prematurely at only 21 years of age. He worked for the radical publisher William Holland and produced powerful anti-slavery material. The cartoon above was in defense of the legal principle of habeas corpus.

Japanese Lithographs Edo Period

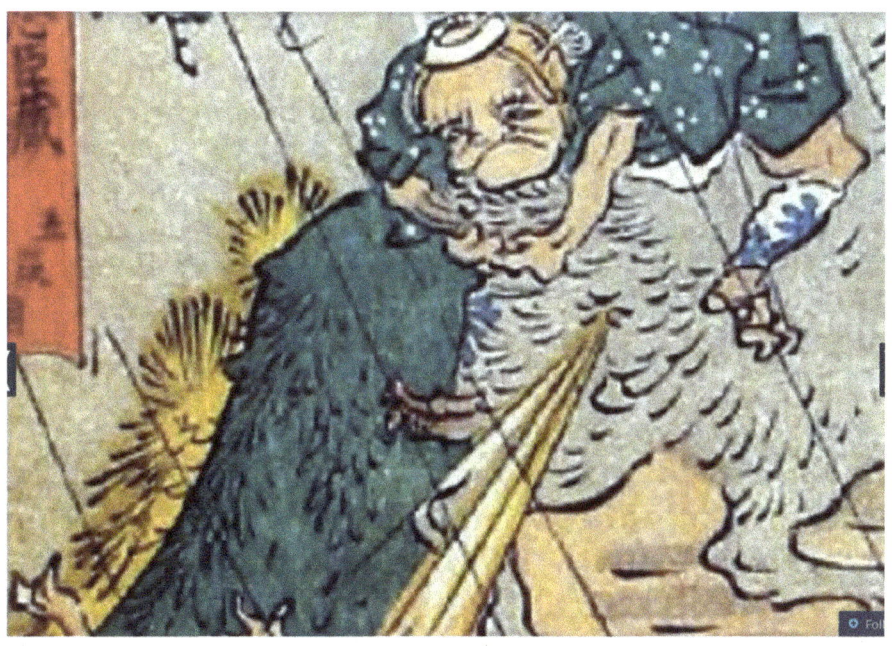

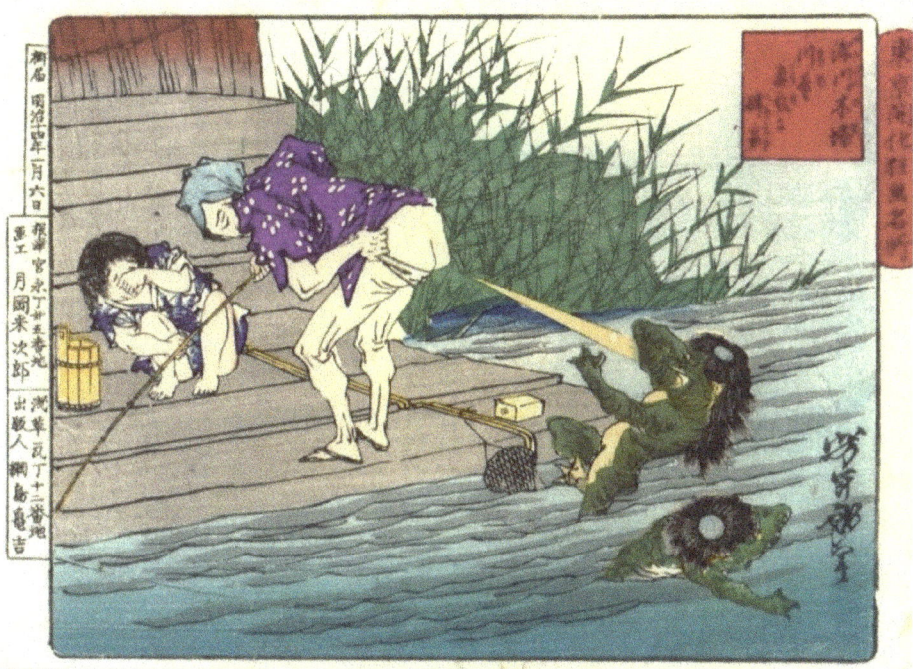

Public Domain

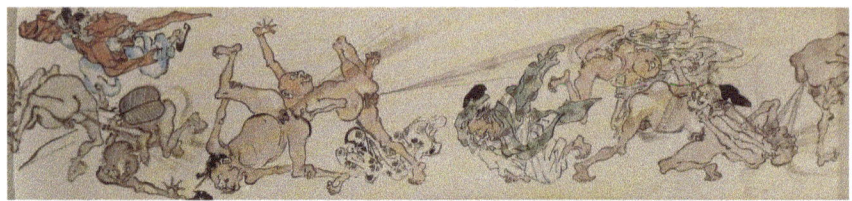

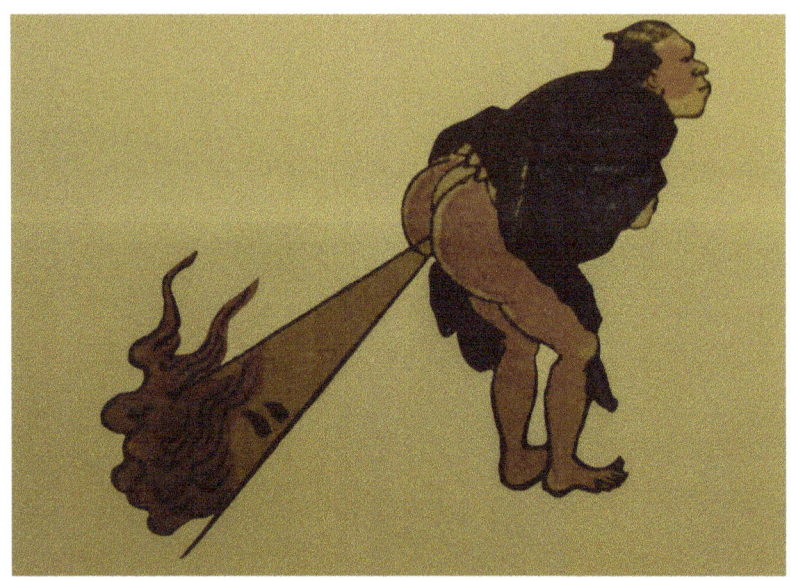

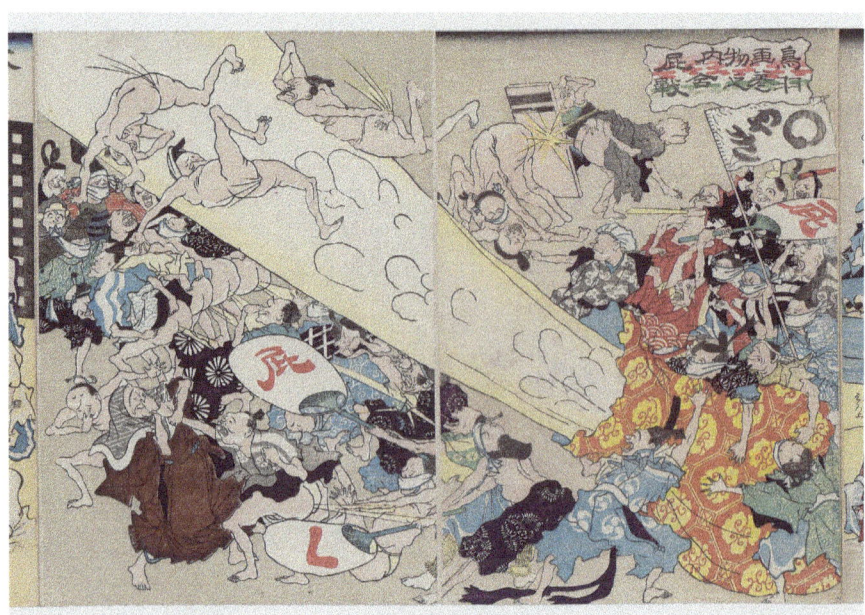

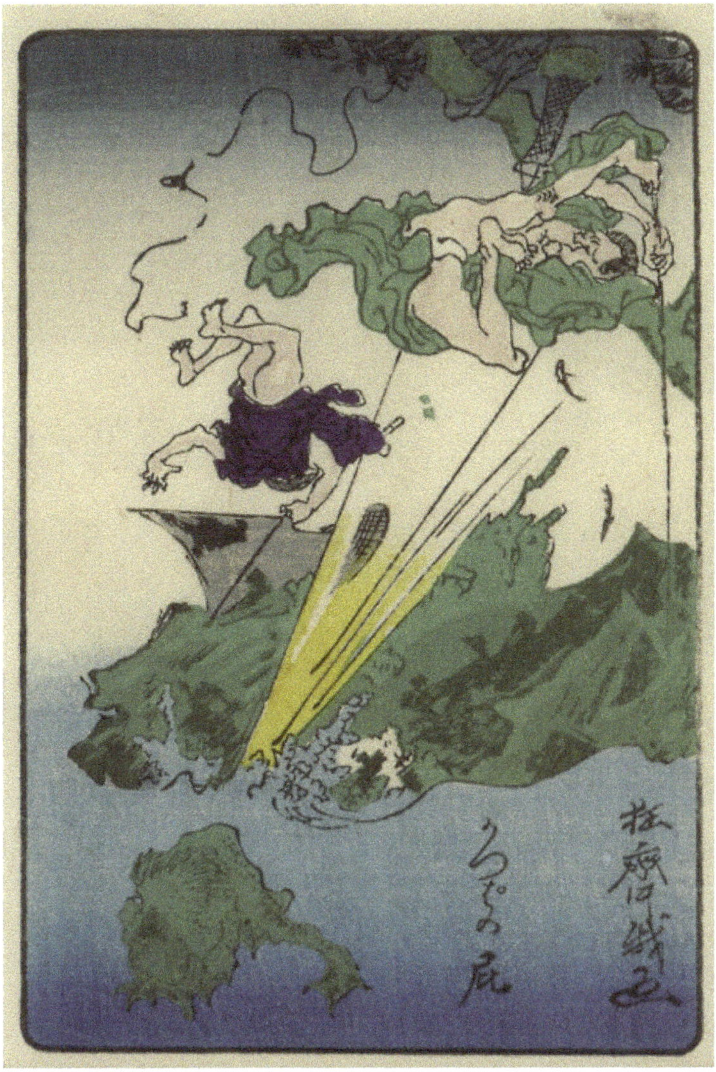

Artsy Fartsy: Cultural History of the Fart Volume One

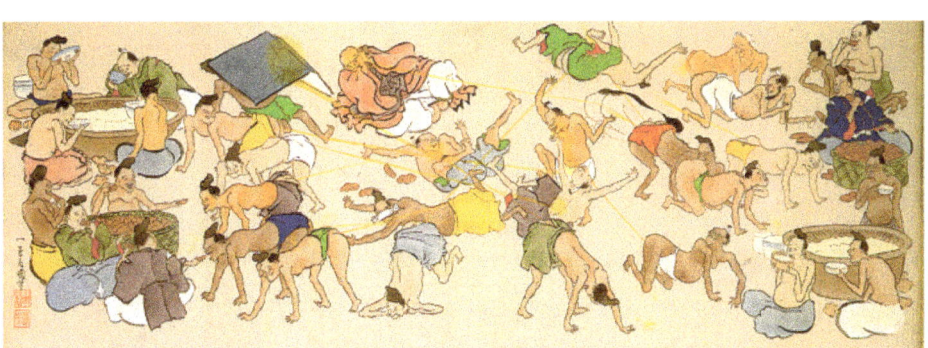

Public Domain

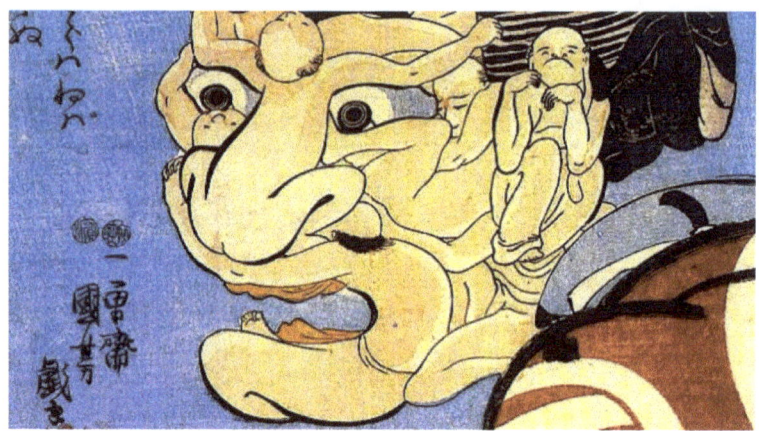
One of Kuniyoshi's composite, butt-nosed paintings (1847-1848)

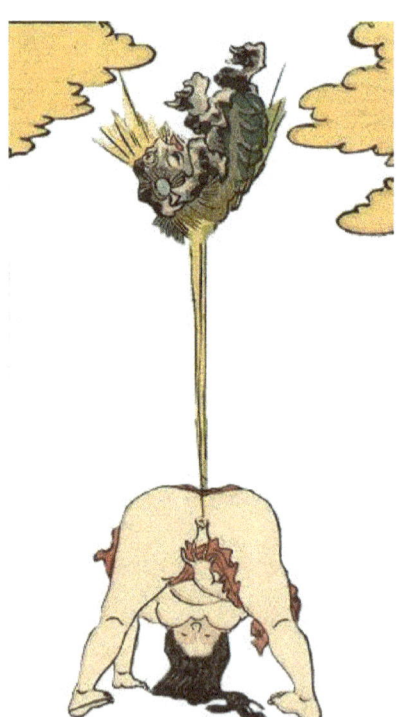
"The fart of a water goblin", kappa no he, 河童の屁, へのかっぱ

The expression "the fart of the water goblin" in Japanese means something small and insignificant. If the water goblin does it in the water, it is not heard very far and does not smell, and very few of us have ever experienced it in real life ... But the real origin of this expression seems to go further, meaning "koppa no hi 木っ端の火", the flame of a little wood splinter used for igniting a fire, which was rather insignificant in itself. People of the Edo period used to play with words, so the KOPPA became a KAPPA.

In Japan a number of individuals earned an income as performers who could utilize their farts for entertainment. This skill set has been prized in other cultures and countries, as described in the entries in this volume on Saint Augustine, Joseph Pujol (Le Pétomane), and Mr. Methane.

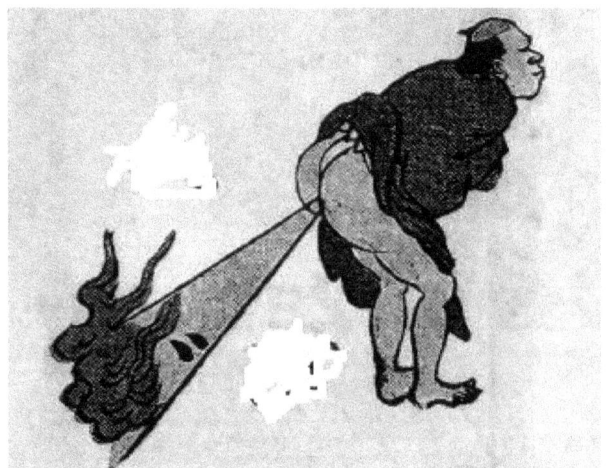

Pun for 蛇 HEBI serpent - he bi to extinguish a fire (hi/bi) with a fart (he)
屁の先に火を描いてヘビ kawasaki-bankin.net

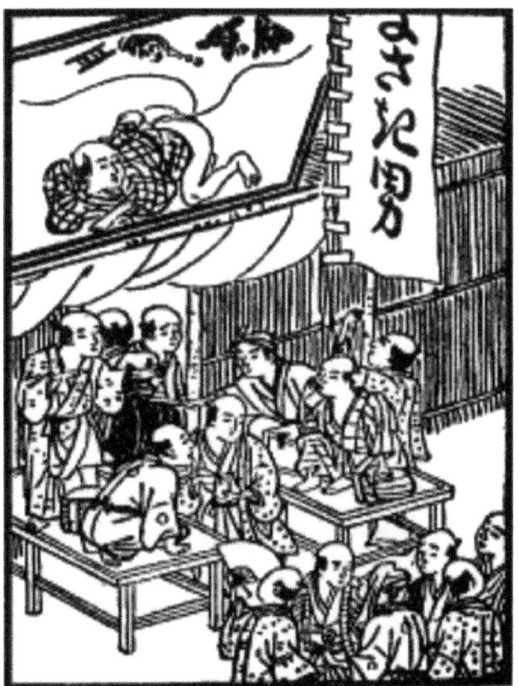

Woodcut illustrating banners over venues with fart entertainment

Utagawa Kuniyoshi (1797 - 1861) was a great master of the popular Japanese Edo Period (1603-1868) ukiyo-e style of woodblock prints and painting. He was an influential member of the Utagawa school. Amongst his many genres he also created Japanese scroll paintings related to farting. The whole scroll from which the images below are taken is called *He-Gassen* (*The Fart Battle*). Original art prints from Utagawa Kuniyoshi are a collectors item. These sell for very high prices on the infrequent occasion when they come up for auction.

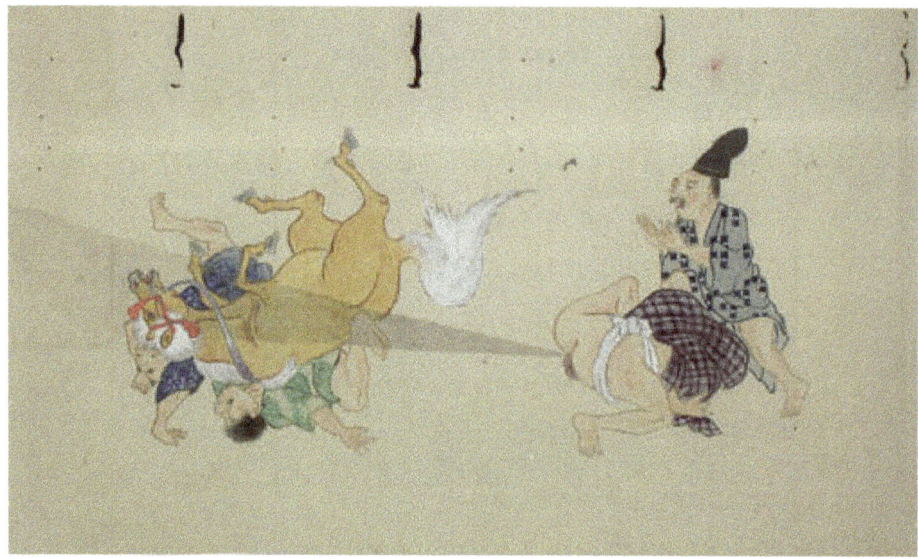

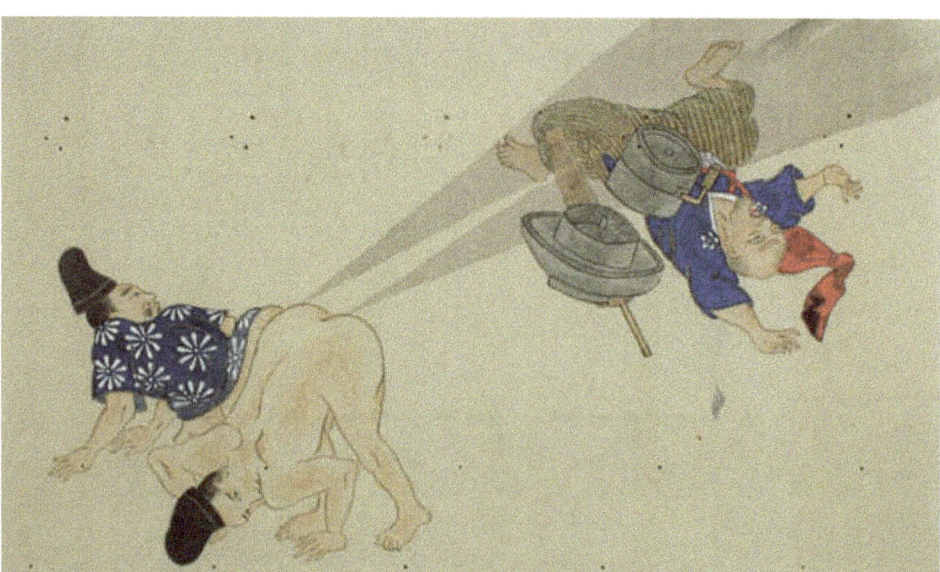

Utagawa Kuniyoshi, Public Domain

Artsy Fartsy: Cultural History of the Fart Volume One

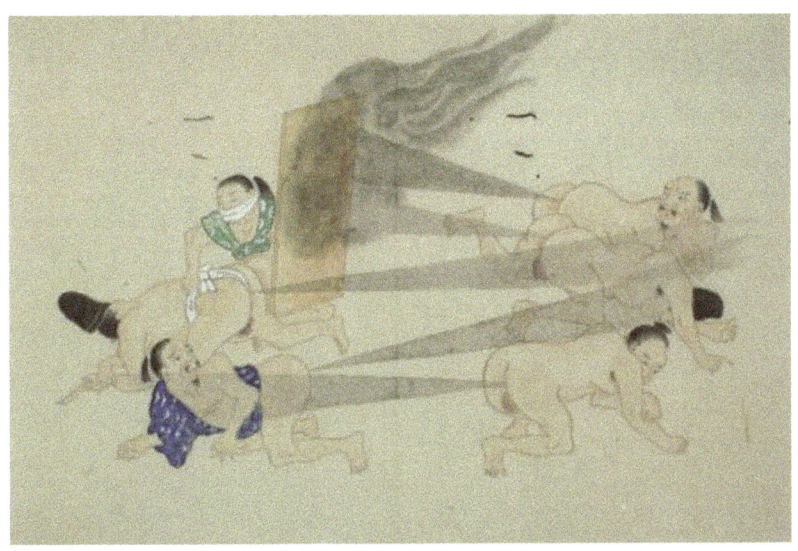

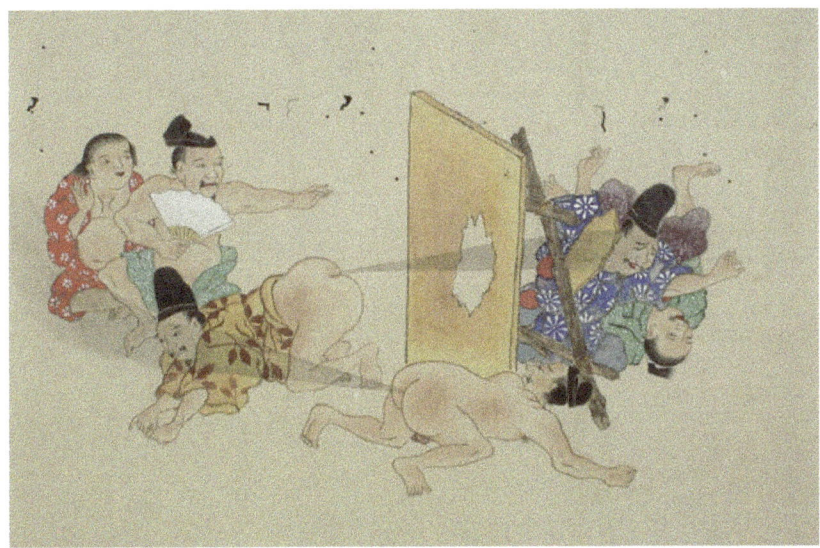

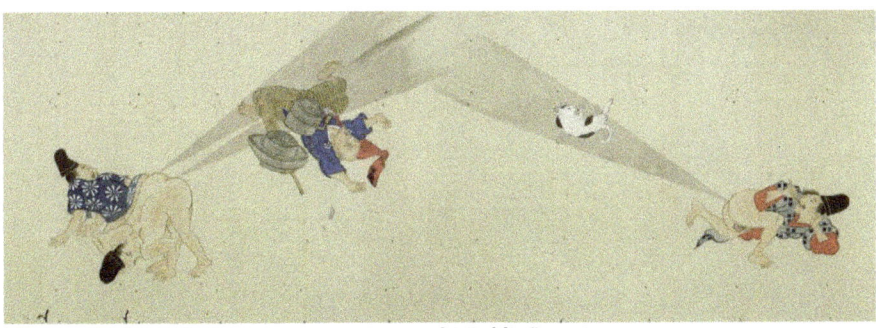

Utagawa Kuniyoshi, Public Domain

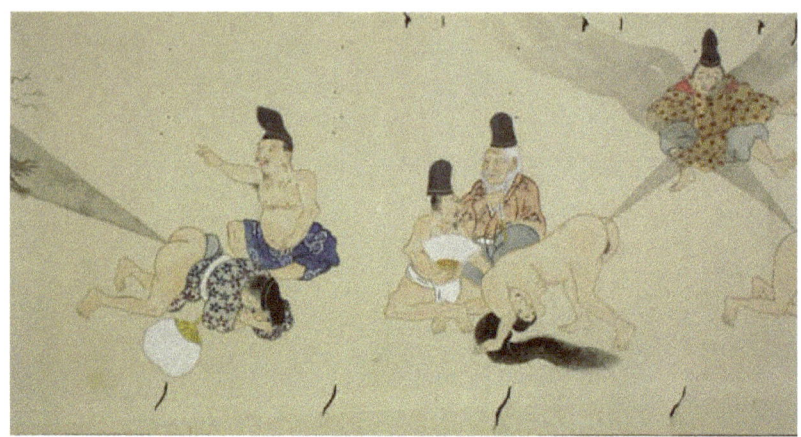
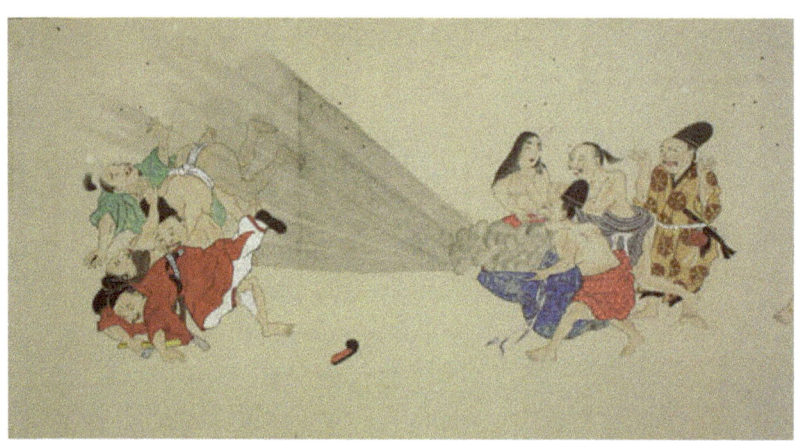
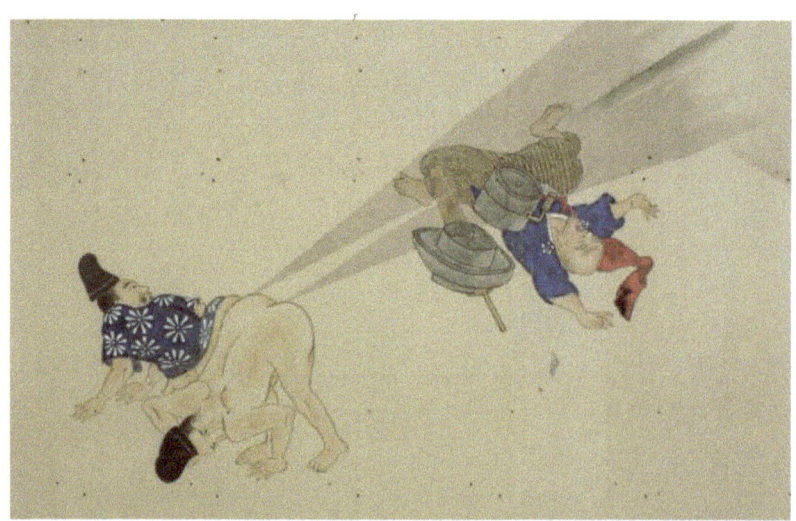

Utagawa Kuniyoshi, Public Domain

Artsy Fartsy: Cultural History of the Fart Volume One

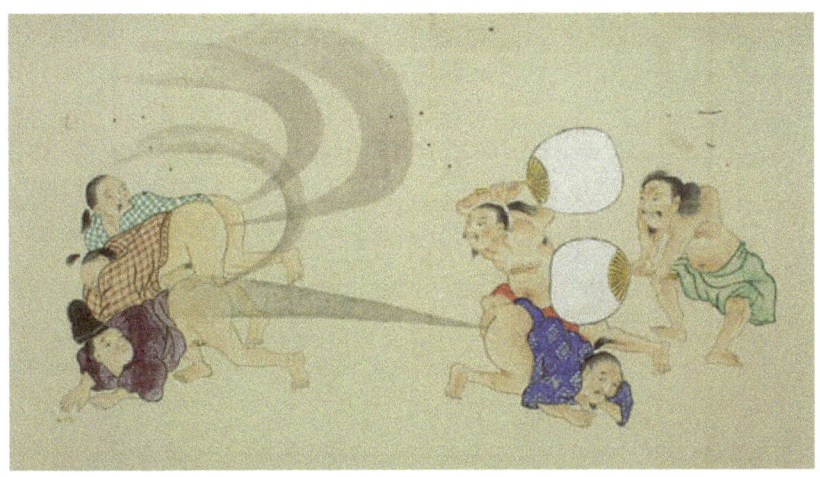

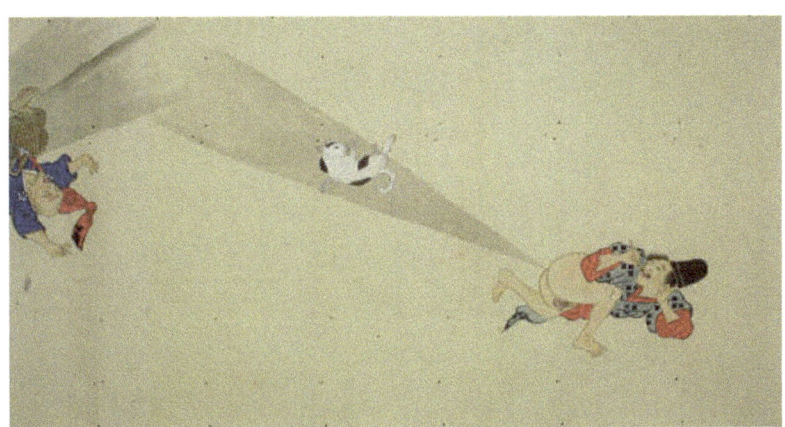

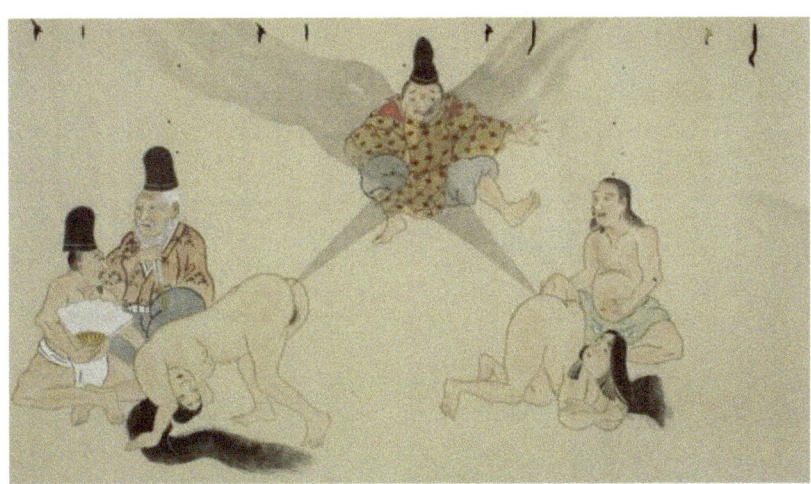

Utagawa Kuniyoshi, Public Domain

Artsy Fartsy: Cultural History of the Fart Volume One

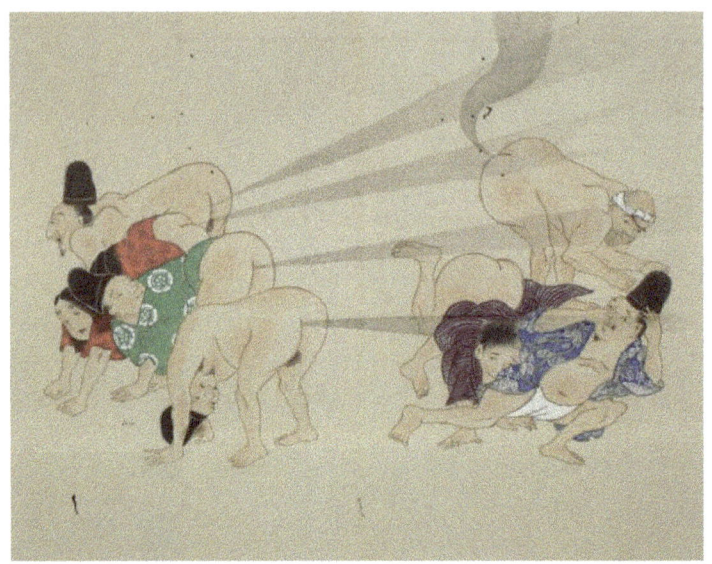

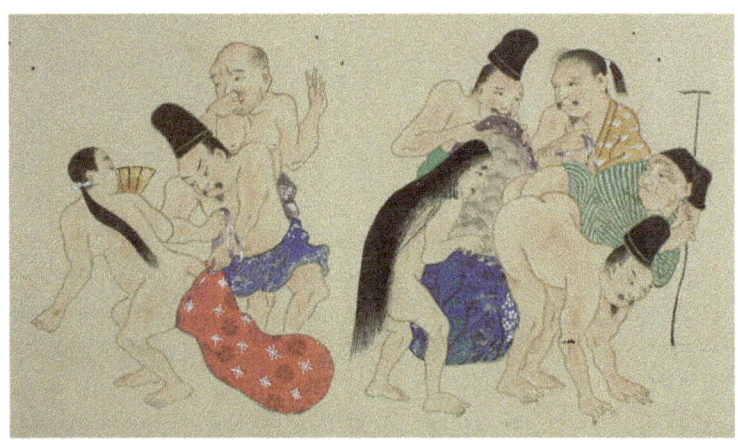

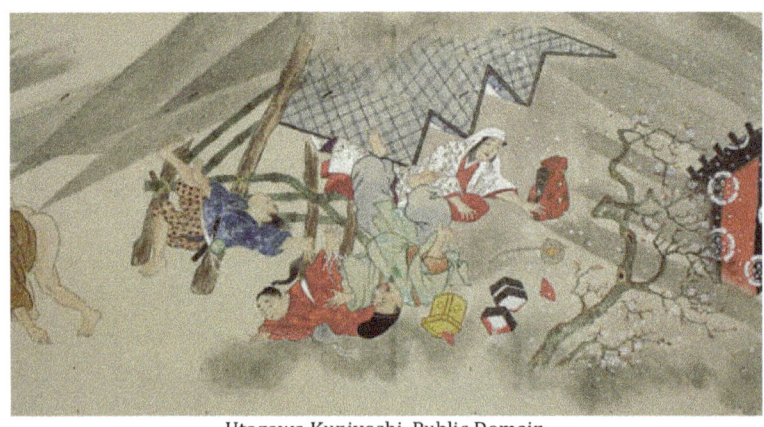

Utagawa Kuniyoshi, Public Domain

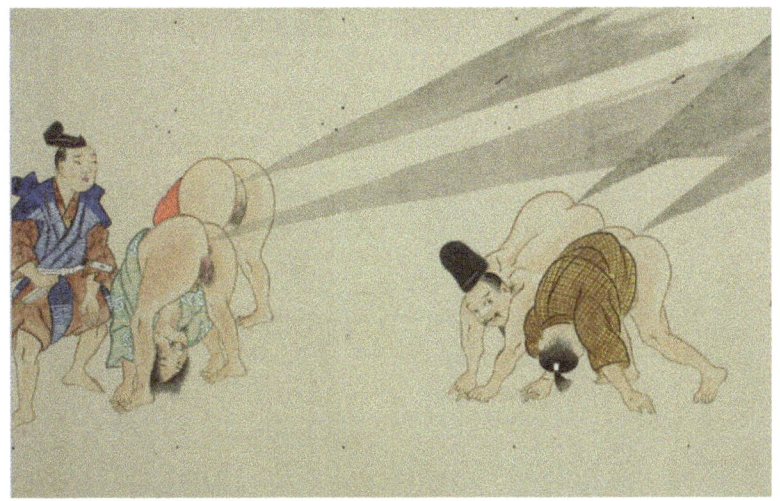
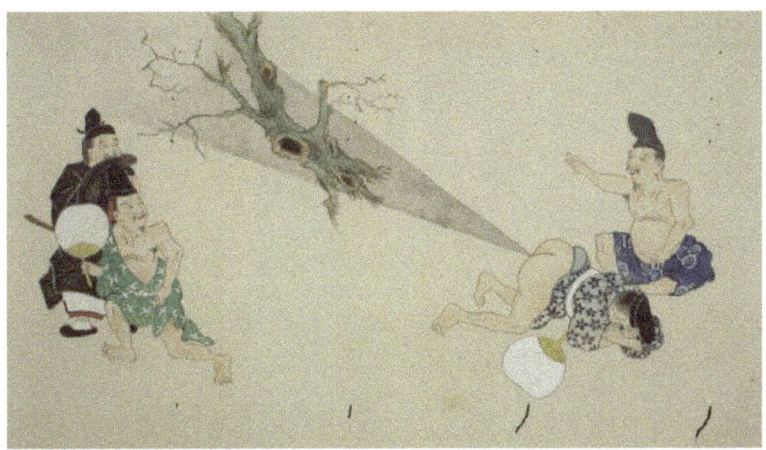
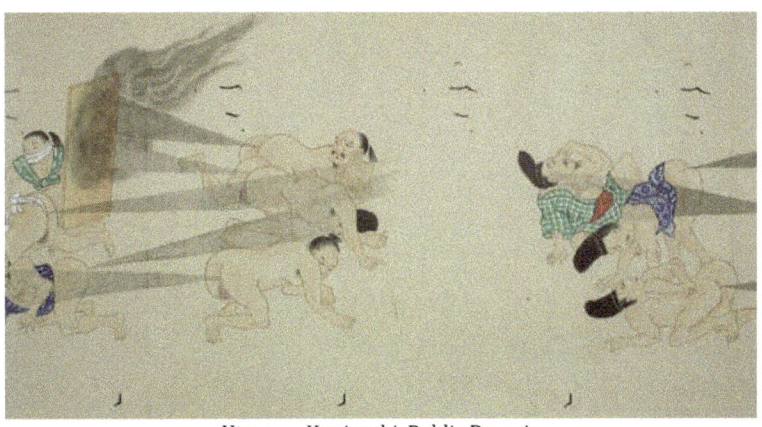

Utagawa Kuniyoshi, Public Domain

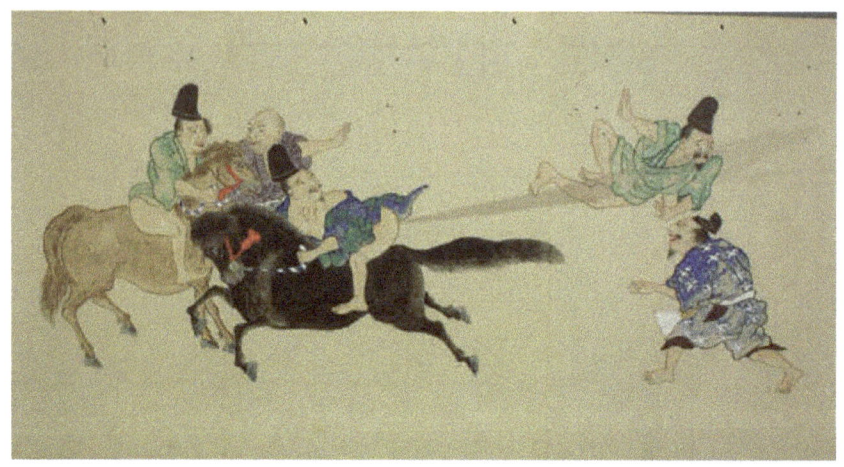

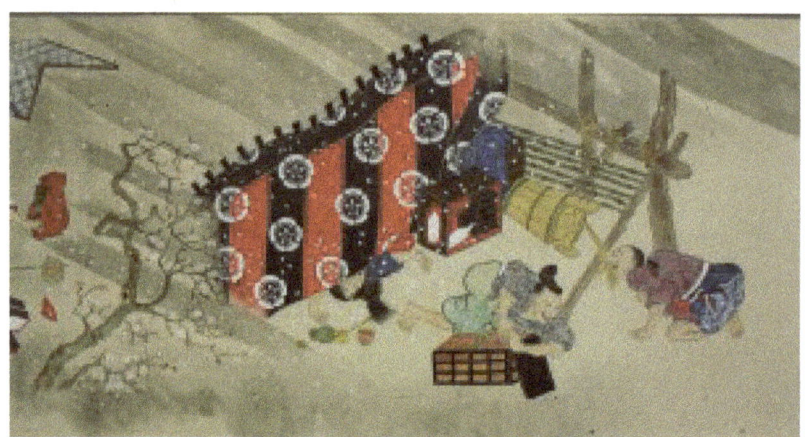

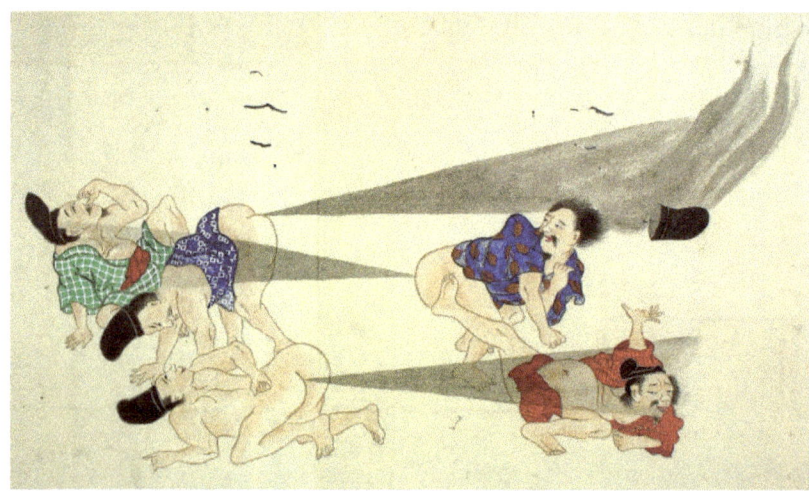

Utagawa Kuniyoshi, Public Domain

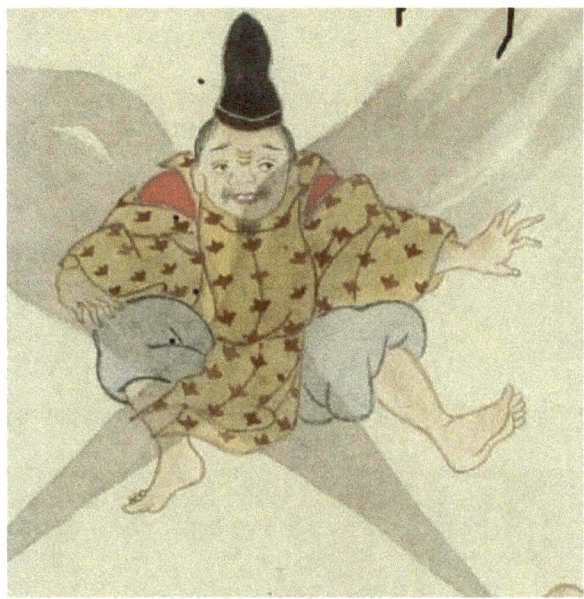
Utagawa Kuniyoshi, Public Domain

George Cruikshank

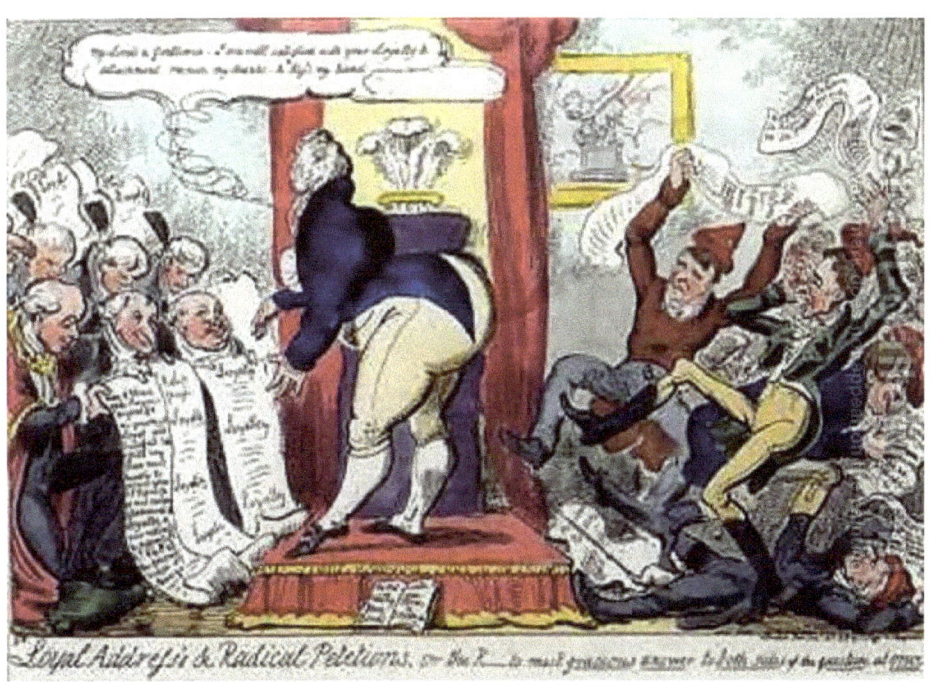
Public Domain

George Cruikshank (1792-1878) was a British caricaturist, illustrator and satirist. He illustrated many of the books of his friends and colleagues including Charles Dickens. He took the place of his major influence, James Gillray, as one of the leading cartoon satirists of his day. In the 1819 image below, the Prince of Wales is farting on his loyal subjects petitioning for reform.

Another caricaturist of the time illustrates an anti-royalist sentiment with a rendition of a game of the times called 'fart-in-the-face". The image depicts Napoleon, King Louis XVIII, and France

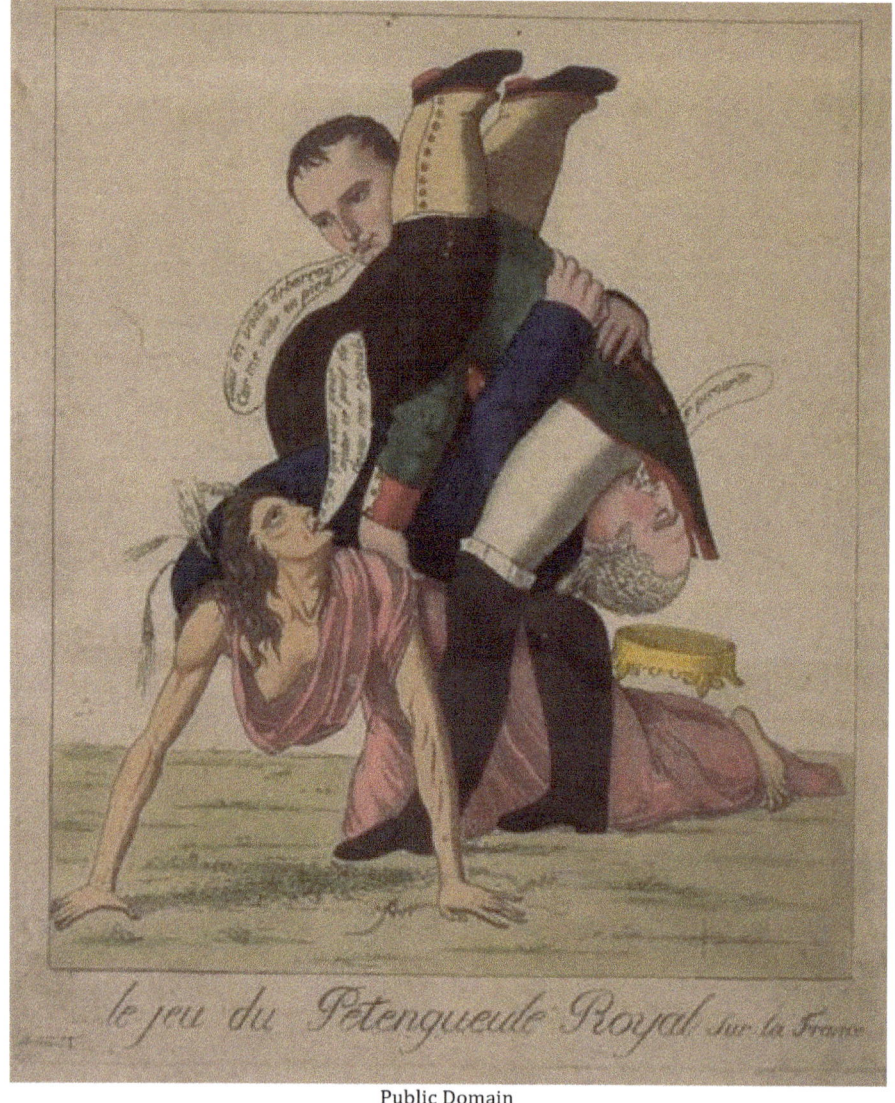

Public Domain

Another scatological image shows Napoleon's field marshal swearing an oath of loyalty just before the Battle of Waterloo.

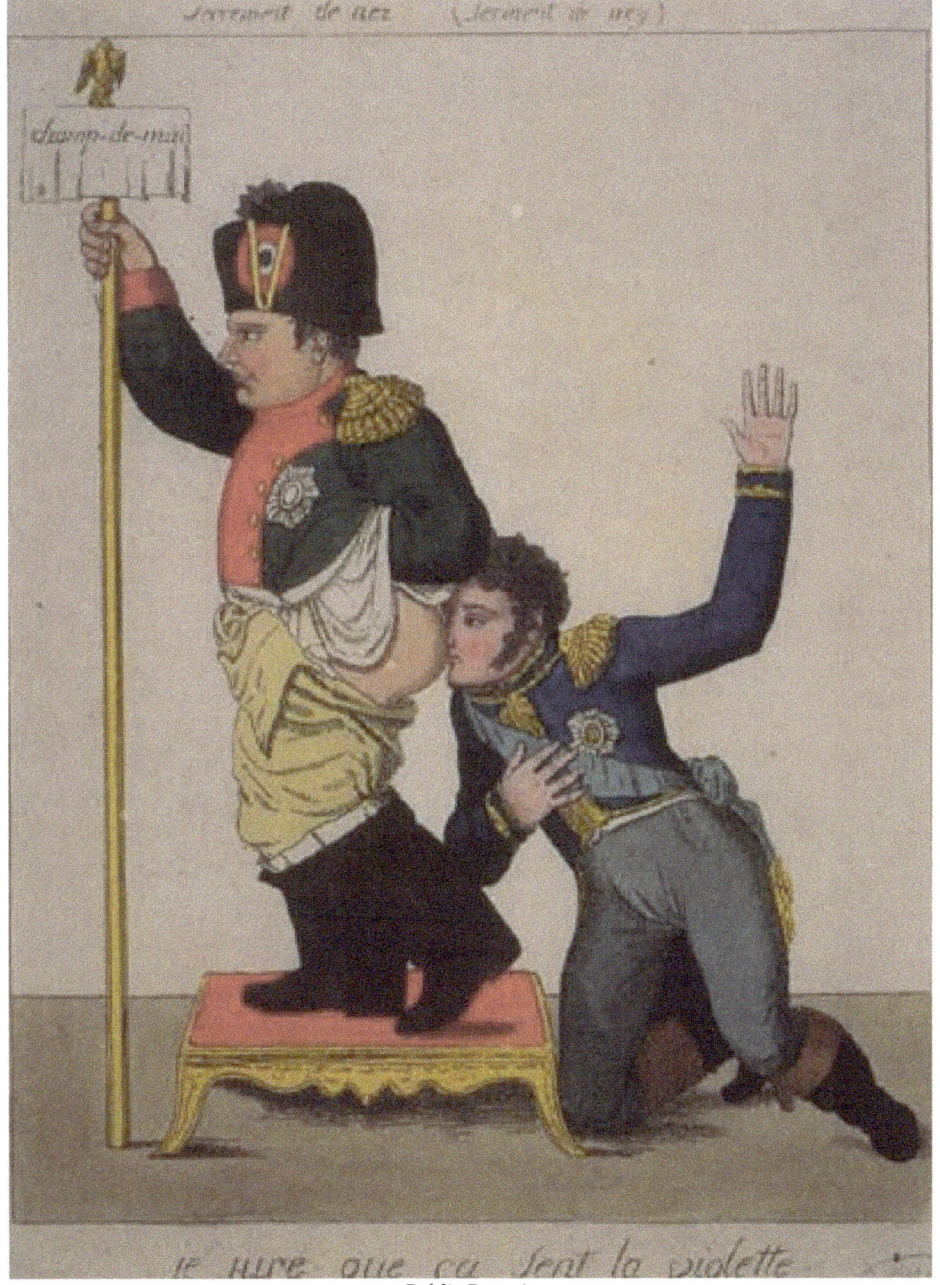

S. Stoutshanks

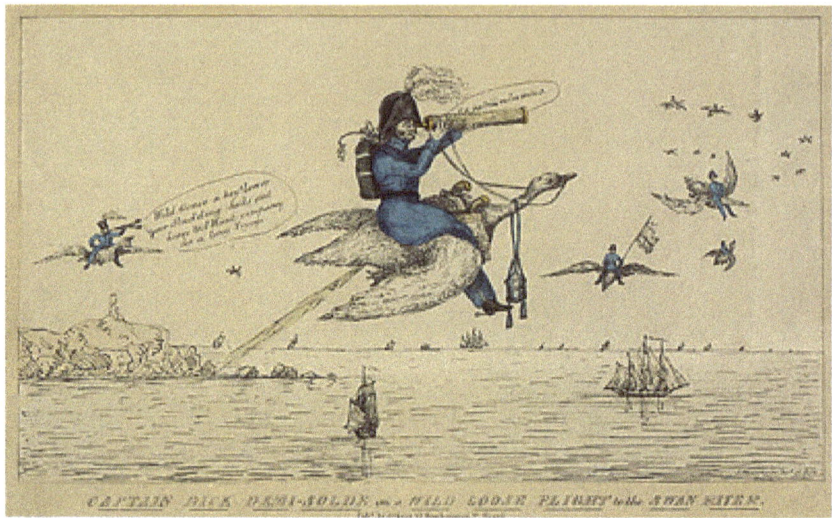

S Stoutshanks 1825 National Gallery of Australia, Public Domain

Stoutshanks was a 19th century cartoonist and illustrator in England active from 1800 to 1830. The lithograph above by Stoutshanks depicts the Duke of Wellington, who was then Prime Minister of England, astride a farting jet propelled white swan. The satirical carton illustrated below criticized a British settlement on the Swan River near Perth Australia.

Richard Wagner

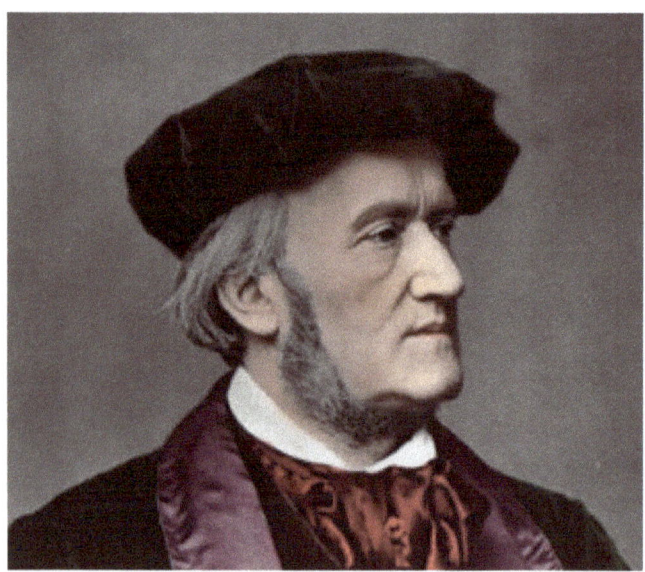

Richard Wagner, Public Domain

Wilhelm Richard Wagner (1813 – 1883) was a German composer, theatre director, and conductor who was best known for his operas. Wagner had his own opera house built, the Bayreuth Festspielhaus.

He had chronic constipation that began in his twenties, and would refer to his lack of productivity both as a digester and composer. He described the "birth of the tetralogy out of the low E flat of flatulence." He regularly complained of flatulence in both directions, referring to his frequent eructation in the same manner as his farts.

He wrote to Carl Landgraf in 1877 complaining in intimate details of hemorrhoids, sluggishness of his unterleib, bloating, and flatulence. To assist his bowels he regularly engaged in colonic irrigations, which although he did not believe helped much, he wrote that they "had become a new religion for me".

Famous Quotations:

"Imagination creates reality."
"Joy is not in things; it is in us."
"Never look at the trombones, it only encourages them."

Aubrey Beardsley

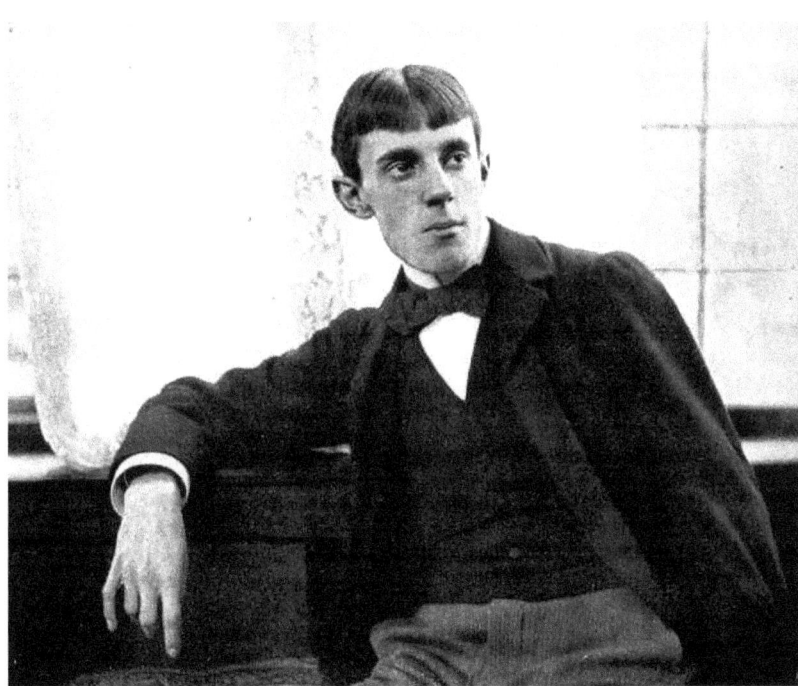

Portrait of English illustrator Aubrey Beardsley (1872 – 1898) by photographer Frederick Hollyer. Public Domain

Aubrey Vincent Beardsley (1872 –1898) was an eccentric English illustrator and author who emphasized the grotesque, the decadent, and the erotic. He said, "I have one aim—the grotesque. If I am not grotesque I am nothing."

His contemporary Oscar Wilde said he had "a face like a silver hatchet, and grass green hair. Poor Aubrey: I hope he will get all right. He brought a strangely new personality to English art, and was a master in his way of fantastic grace, and the charm of the unreal. His muse had moods of terrible laughter. Behind his grotesques there seemed to lurk some curious philosophy..." Despite a premature death from tuberculosis at the age of twenty-six he made significant contributions to the artistic style of Art Nouveau and posters.

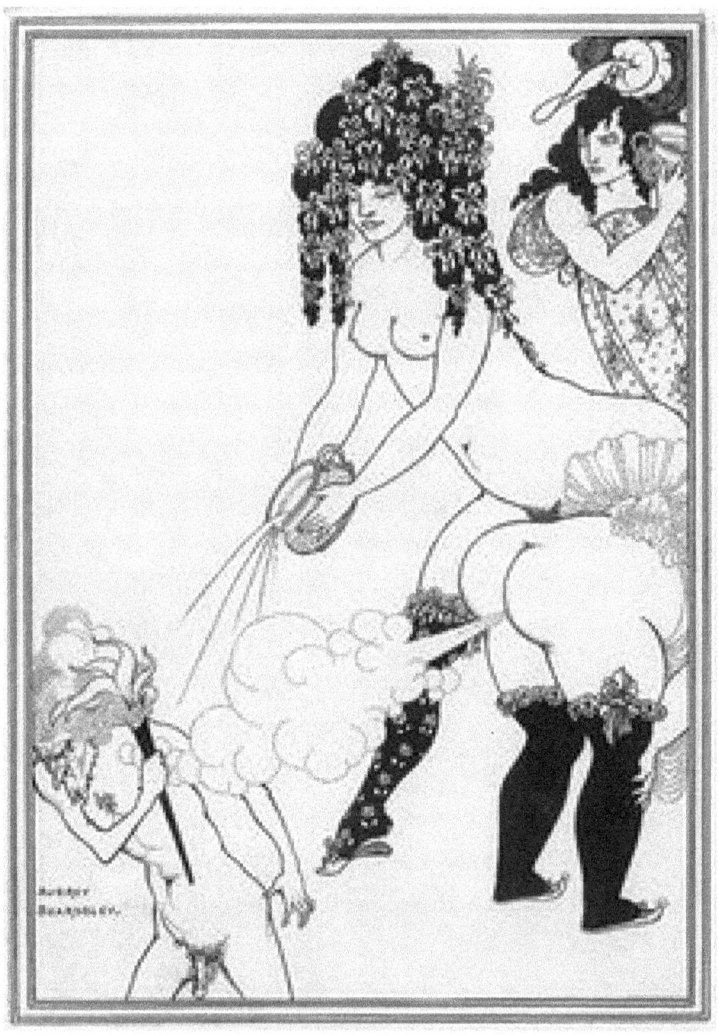

Lysistrata Defending the Acropolis, by Aubrey Beardsley, Public Domain

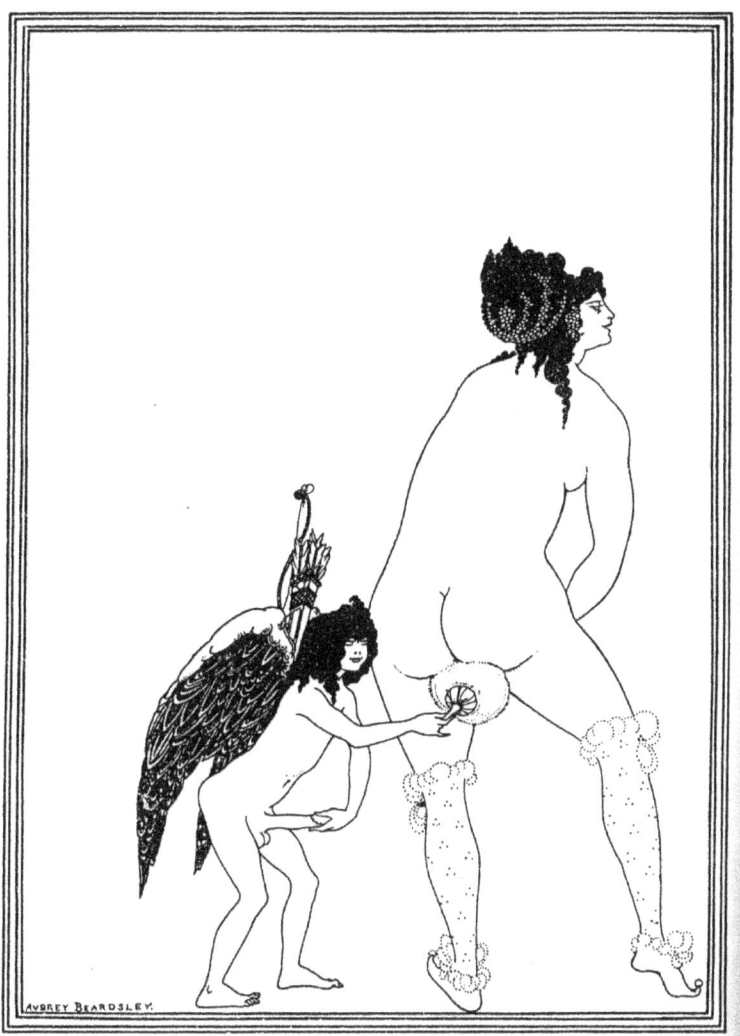

Joseph Pujol (Le Pétomane)

Joseph Pujol (1857 – 1945) was a stage performer from 1887 to 1914, and first performed on the Moulin Rouge stage in Paris in 1892. He had the unusual ability to inhale air into his colon through his anus and expel it at will. With the stage name Le Pétomane, French for the fart maniac, he was also affectionately known as 'the fartiste'.

With sufficient colonic inhalations and exhalations he was able to minimize the odor and control the sounds emanating from his anus to such a degree that he could play musical tunes. To assure that there was no odor he also underwent regular colonic irrigations before performances.

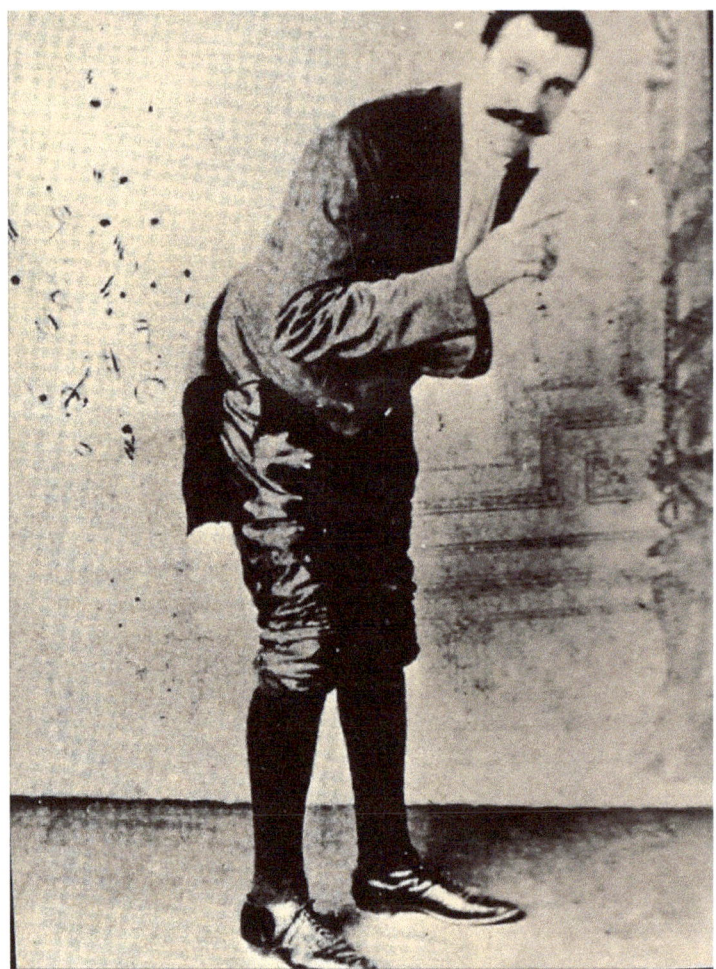

Joseph Pujol (Le Pétomane) 1857, Public Domain

Appearing on stage in red cape, white cravat, and black trousers, with a pair of white gloves held in the hands, he displayed the incongruous touch of elegance that added to his charm. A program of fart impressions followed, including contrasting the hearty fart of the miller with the timid fart of the young girl.

He proceeded to demonstrate the diffidence of the fart of the bride on her wedding night (almost inaudible) compared to the fart of the bride a week later (a lusty raspberry). His musical impersonations included an imitation of a tuba player on his instrument. He stunned the audience with a majestic ten-second fart, which he likened to a couturier cutting six feet of calico cloth.

He would play *Le Marseilles* on his personal human wind instrument, his colon, even though he could only produce four notes do, mi, so, and the octave do. To add to his musical repertoire he would insert a tube offstage into his rectum and attach it to the musical instrument the ocarina. Then playing *O' Sole Mio* he would invite the audience to sing along.

Replacing the musical instrument at the end of the tube with a cigarette he used his colon to inhale. After withdrawal of the tube he would exhale the cigarette smoke out of his behind. For the grand finale he would imitate a twenty-one-gun salute, and the Great 1906 San Francisco earthquake with a thunderous roar that went on for over five continuous minutes. He would end his performance by blowing out a candle at a distance of three feet.

Other than Harry Houdini, he was the highest paid stage performer in Europe and was earning a salary of twenty thousand francs per week. This was substantially more than the eight thousand francs per week salary of his contemporary Sarah Bernhardt who was considered the leading lady of the stage at that time. King Leopold II of Belgium and Edwards Prince of Wales came incognito to see Le Pétomane perform. Sigmund Freud attended a performance, and perhaps inspired, went on to describe his theory of anal fixation.

At one point he was embroiled in a disagreement with his stage manager and was going to perform in a different venue. The manager went to the courts and got a judicial injunction preventing Le Pétomane from performing elsewhere. During the court hearing Le Pétomane demonstrated his unique abilities in front of the court (he judge did not rule him out of order, or in contempt of court). Le Pétomane decided to offer his farting services and performance for free in a public display, but the manager and the court decision forbade him to fart in public.

When he died, the physicians of the day wanted to do a postmortem examination to find out how he had such remarkable anal control. The family held onto his body until enough decomposition set in that they no longer had to fear grave robbers retrieving the body for science. Joseph Pujol's memorable life lives on in the cinematic and stage arts. In Mel Brooks' 1974 movie Blazing Saddles, with many memorable fart scenes, there is an inside joke. It is an artistic acknowledgement to Joseph Pujol with Mel Brooks himself playing Governor William LePetomane.

James Ensor

James Ensor was an international celebrity whose art baffled viewers with psychological complexity, internal contradictions, and eccentricity. The colored etching below called *Doctrinal Nourishment* shows the highest leaders of 1800s European society — a king, a cardinal, a general and a judge — squatting bare-bummed as they defecate into the wide-open mouths of their supine, passive subjects. His scandalous artwork gave him notoriety and acclaim in his native Belgium and beyond.

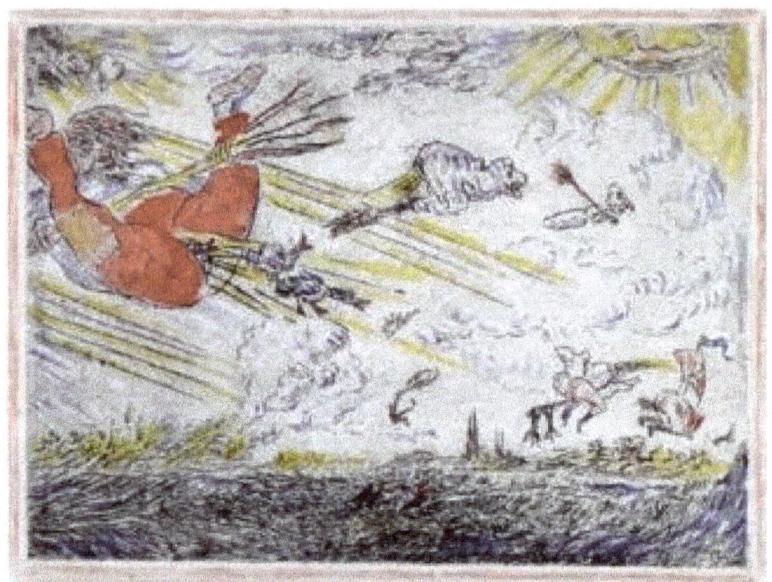

James Ensor, Wizards in a Squall, Public Domain

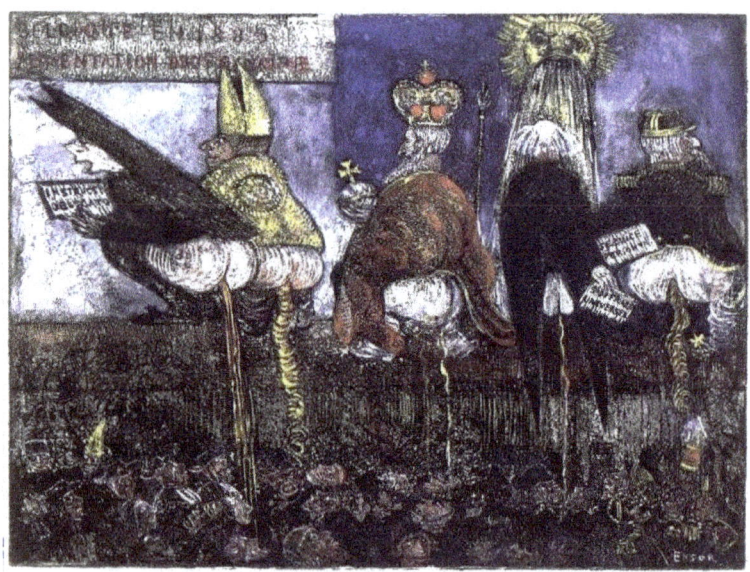

James Ensor, Doctrinal Nourishment www.scpr.org Creative Commons License

Famous Quotations:

"Reason and nature are the enemy of the artist."
"Drenched in British purples, I have offered up my tones: pigeon breast, hind belly, balky mule lung, monkey bottom pink, lapis lazuli and malachite, excited nymph thigh, panther pee-pee, high-smelling hen hair, hedgehog in aspic, barrel-

maker's brothel, revered rose, monkeybush, turkey-like white, sly violet, page's slipper, immaculate nun spring, unspeakable red, Ensor azure, affected yellow, mummy skull, rock-hard gray, brunt celadon, shop soiled smoke ring."

Canadian Broadcast Corporation

Attributed to the staff of the Canadian Broadcast Corporation in the 1940's, a record called *The Crepitation Contest* was produced. Canadian Broadcast Corporation sportscaster Sidney S. Brown narrated it, with sound effects credited to his producer, Jules Lipton. The recording is a parody of a radio broadcast of a live sporting event with pre-game interviews of the contestants.

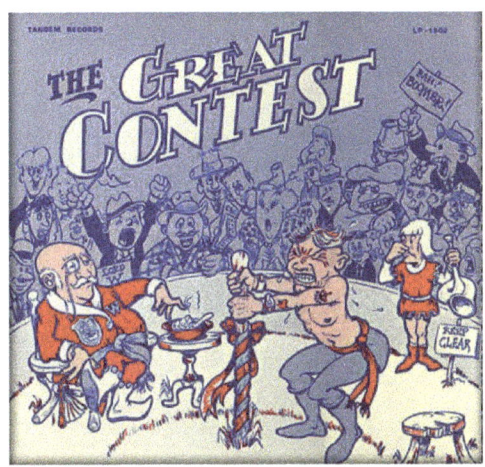

www.wfmu.org Creative Commons License

The reigning champion is Lord Windesmear and the challenger is Paul Boomer. The broadcast parody includes detailed descriptions of the competition including the rules, traditions, play-by-play reporting if the event and audience sounds and reactions.

Reportedly the original recording was played at a New Year's Eve party in 1943 that was attended by an admiral of the United States Navy. He believed it would be a great morale booster for American serviceman. The original master recording at RCA Victor's studio in Toronto was obtained and lacquer and vinyl 78-rpm discs were pressed.

Salvador Dali

Salvador Domingo Felipe Jacinto Dalí i Domènechl (1904 – 1989) was an eccentric, colorful, and prominent Spanish surrealist painter born in Figueres, in the Catalonia region of Spain. His autobiography entitled *The Secret Life of Salvador Dali* was posthumously published in 1993. He openly discusses his lifelong fascination and obsession with farts.

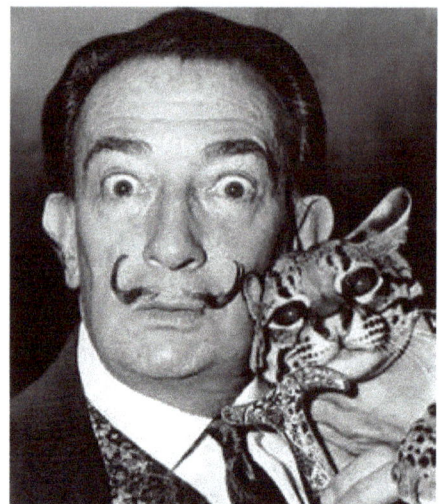

Salvador Dali with ocelot and cane 1965 Author Robert Higgins New York World-Telegram & Sun Collection, Public Domain

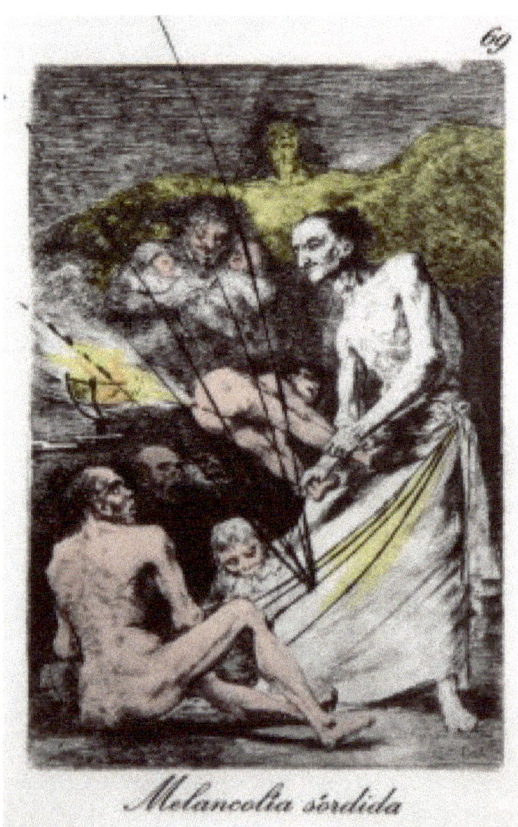

Dali -Sopla Gust the wind Capricho 1977 Based on Francisco Goya's etchings

Famous Quotations:

"Have no fear of perfection - you'll never reach it."
 "I don't do drugs. I am drugs."
 "Intelligence without ambition is a bird without wings."
"A true artist is not one who is inspired, but one who inspires others."
 "The only difference between me and a madman is I'm not mad."
"I am not strange. I am just not normal."
"One day it will have to be officially admitted that what we have christened reality is an even greater illusion than the world of dreams."
"There is only one difference between a madman and myself. The madman thinks he is sane. I know I am mad."

Cinematic Arts

Farts have been in movies from the very beginning, you just did not know it because they were silent films. It was said that Rudolph Valetino, the suave leading man of many romantic silent films, was notorious for his extensive fart emanations on the film stage.

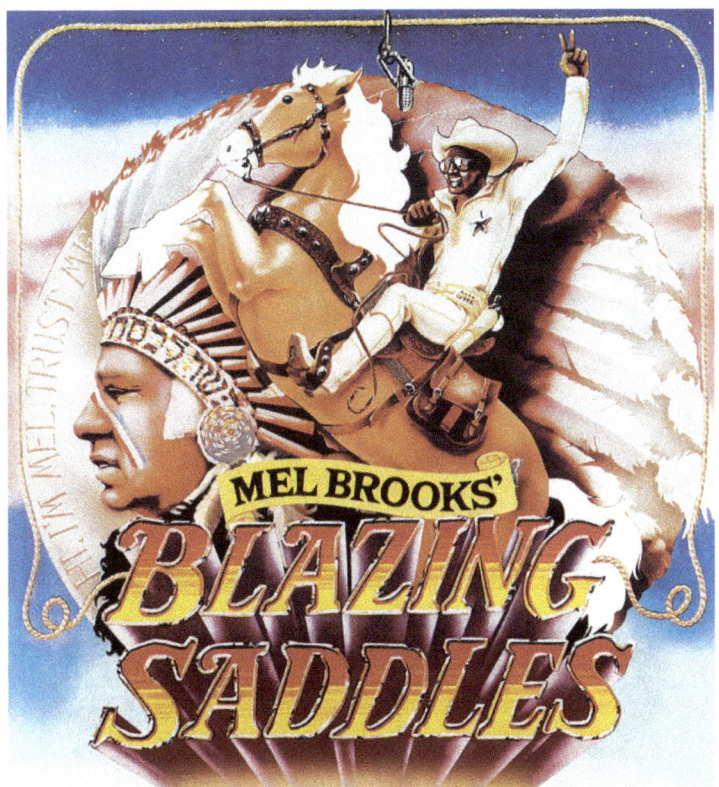

mr-darko-movie-log.blogspot.com Creative Commons License

Artsy Fartsy: Cultural History of the Fart Volume One

The secret of cinematic farts has been out of the bag for a long time, especially since the classic fart marathon of Mel Brook's *Blazing Saddles*. The character he plays, Governor Pétomane is so named in honor of the famous Frenchman, Joseph Pujol, who brought farting to the heights of the entertainment world on Paris' famous Moulin Rouge (see entry on Joseph Pujol).

In 2013 the American Film Institute recognized the fart trail Mel Brooks blazed by bestowing on him its 41st Life Achievement Award. As Sir Howard Stringer, the CEO of Sony Pictures and the chair of the AFI Board of Trustees announced to the star studded banquet: "Ladies and gentleman, tonight the American Film Institute honors the arts, and the farts, of American film".

Another memorable fart quote is from Monty Python. "I don't want to talk to you no more, you empty headed animal food trough wiper. I fart in your general direction. Your mother was a hamster and your father smelt of elderberries." — Graham Chapman, *Monty Python and the Holy Grail*

Besides the cinematic arts, farts have become common fodder for television, radio, and other forms of media communication. The advent of the Internet, video clips such as YouTube, and virtually unlimited access to distribute content from individuals has led to a veritable explosion of farts in media.

The Nutty Professor
Blazing Saddles
Step Brothers
Dumb and Dumber
Ghost World
The Sopranos
South Park: Bigger, Longer & Uncut
Dances with Wolves
Rain Man
Amadeus
Biloxi Blues
Transformers: Beast Wars
Jay and Silent Bob Strike Back
Shrek
Airplane!
Mystery Men
Dances with Wolves
Shaun of the Dead
Beavis and Butthead
Caddyshack
South Park
Blazing Saddles
Henry Fool
Dumb and Dumber

Tideland
A Prairie Home Companion
A Clockwork Orange
Master of Disguise
Satyricon
Good Morning
35 Shots of Rum
Amarcord
Control
King Lear: Fear and Loathing
Fanny and Alexander
Ohayo
Stroszek
Y Tu Mama Tambien
Harry Potter 3
Children of Men
La Grande Bouffe
Kabei, Our Mother
Volver
Wertmuller's Seven Beauties
Shaun Of The Dead
The Madness of King George
10
Fanny and Alexander
Rango
The Lion King
Blazing Saddles
Last King of Scotland
South Park
The Nutty Professor
Rocketman
The Man
Click
Austin Powers Goldmember
Tenacious D In the Pick of Destiny
I Love You Man
Year One
Step Brothers
Extreme Movie
Hall Pass
Scooby Doo
Josh
Along Came Polly
Dennis the Menace
Scary Movie
Grumpy Old Men

Pink Panther
Fartin Gary & Fartin Rudy
The Fatties
Ghost World
The Sopranos
South Park: Bigger, Longer, & Uncut
Finding Nemo
Transformers: Beast Wars
Twilight
Funny People
My Best Friends Girl
Knocked Up
Love and Other Disasters
Ten Canoes
Idiocracy
The Departed
Life on Mars
Larry the Cable Guy, Health Inspectors
Ace Ventura
Hannah Montana
The Man
Doctor Who
Once Upon a Time In Mexico
The Venture Brothers
Monk
Moonlight Mile
15 Storeys High
Popworld
Grim and Evil
Jay and Silent Bob Strike Back
Chump Change
Last Action Hero
Spies Like Us
Harold and Kumar Go To White Castle
Can't Buy Me Love
Police Academy
American Pie
Mystery Men
Men in Black
Naked Gun
Hot Shots Part Deux
Brain Donors
Austin Powers International Man of Mystery
The Heartbreak Kid
Bigger
The Hollywood Knights

Artsy Fartsy: Cultural History of the Fart Volume One

Black Sheep
Six-shooter
Liar, Liar
Mean Girls
Thunderpants
F.A.R.T. The Movie
The Usual Suspects
The Whole Nine Yards
Carpool
Simpsons
Seinfeld
The Interview

Bollywood Hindi Movies

Movies, film, and television have an international appeal and marketplace. The movie industry has a second capital to compete with Hollywood. Based in Mumbai, India, a city that was known in the past as Bombay, the new capital has the nickname Bollywood.

The movies from Bollywood are not limited in their appeal to speakers of Hindi, and have an international following. A number of them have become major award winners as well as financial blockbusters. The blogger rohit-ghosh.blogspot.com has written extensively about the impact of the fart on the movie capital of India, Bollywood.

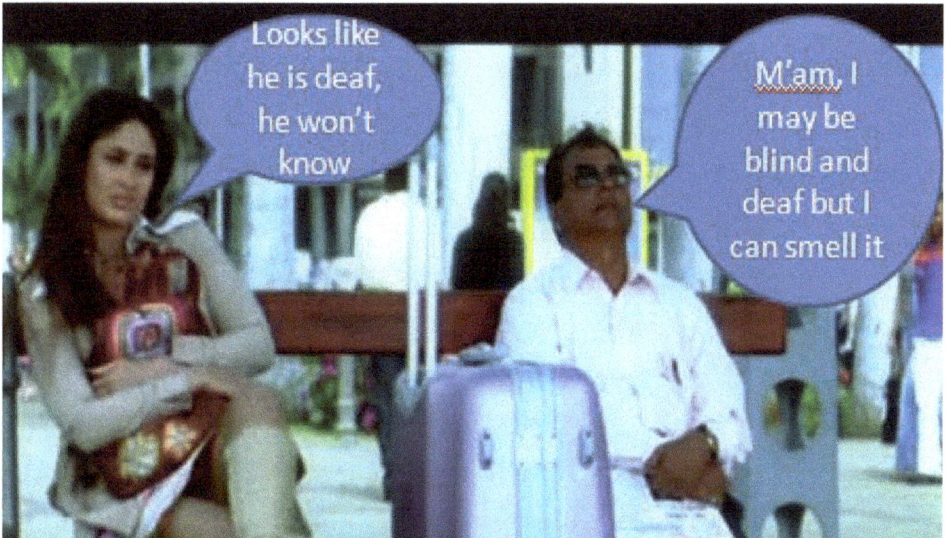

www.zimbio.com Creative Commons License

Seinfeld

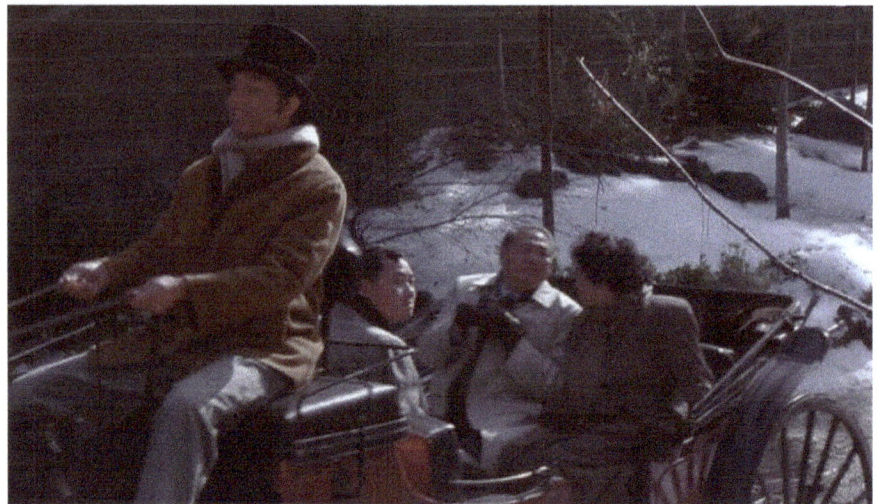

Seinfeld episode with horse farts www.youtube.com/watch?v=lroZLN1gQnw

The well-known phenomenon of horse farts have been exploited on television with an episode of the comedy series *Seinfeld* entitled *The Rye*. Cramer feeds the horse a beef and pasta meal pulling a hansom carriage in Central Park in New York City. It makes the horse so extremely flatulent so that Cramer and the passengers in the carriage cannot bear the gas exposure.

Mr. Methane

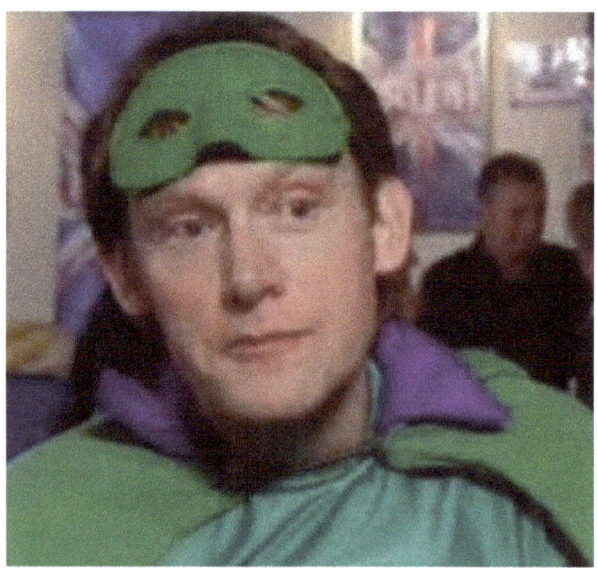

Mr. Methane (Paul Oldfield) world-rising-entertainment.blogspot.com Creative Common License

Mr. Methane (Paul Oldfield) (1966-) is a British comedy stage performer who claims to be the world's only flatulist, a professional farter. He states that he discovered his ability at age fifteen while practicing yoga (see separate entry on yoga), and performed for his friends the following day. He has been performing ever since, attempting to emulate the stage success of Le Pétomane (Joseph Pujol).

He has performed on *Britain's Got Talent* to a mixture of harsh criticism and laughter from the judges, especially Simon Cowell who was not amused. He has also released flatulent recordings of his parody performances of songs, often to hostile reception from the original artists.

Budweiser Super Bowl Commercial

An equine fart theme took place in a prime and extremely expensive Super Bowl advertisement for Budweiser beer. A man and a young woman are in a romantic horse drawn carriage. He presents her with a lit candle and reaches down to pull up some bottles of Budweiser beer.

As he is bending over and out of the way getting the beer the horse's tail lifts. The horse farts and the candle explodes in a ball of flame obscuring the young woman's facial features. When the man sits back upright he smells smoke and asks if she smells a barbeque.

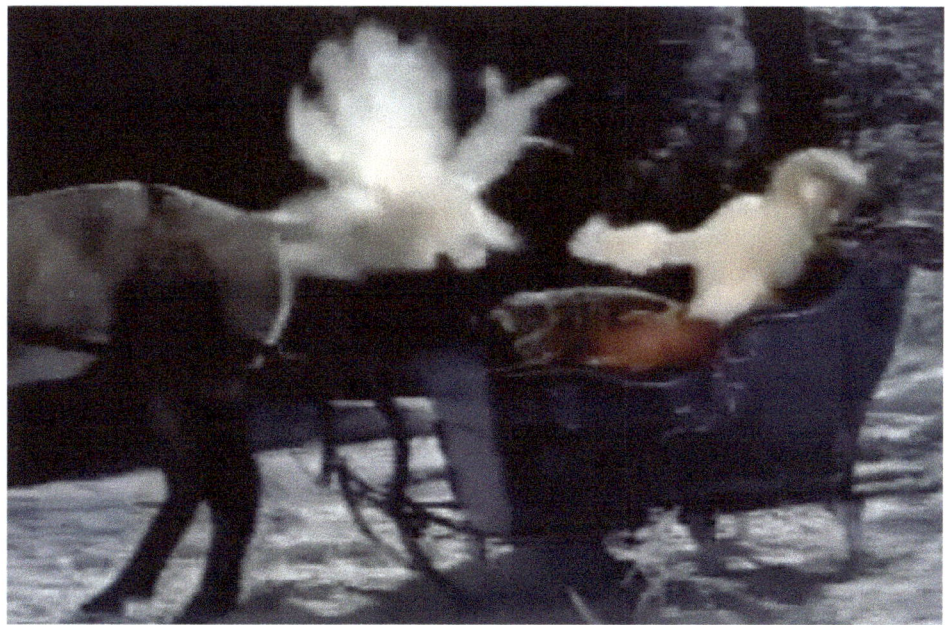

www.youtube.com/watch?v=FhaYvI1yrUM

The Lion King

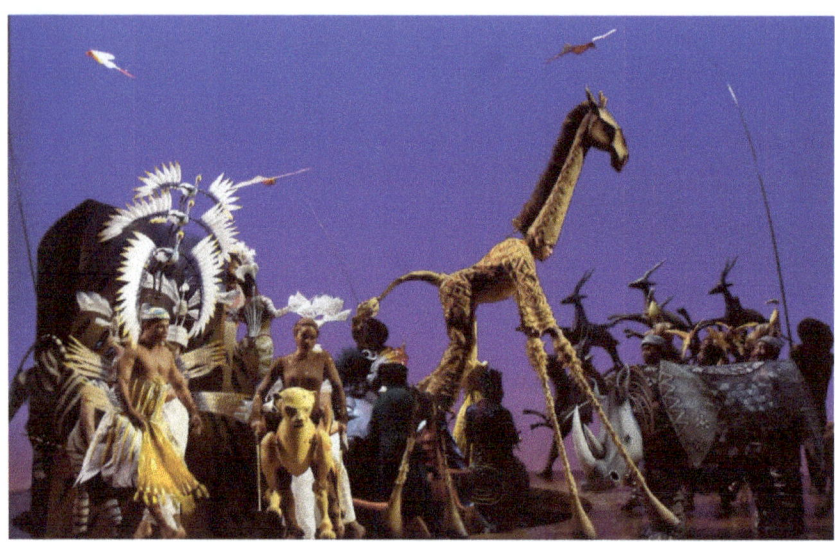

The Lion King Musical www.galleryhip.com

The Lion King was a very successful award winning animated motion picture produced by Walt Disney Studios. The score was composed by Sir Elton John and the lyrics by Tim Rice. It was subsequently transferred to the live stage as a musical under the direction of Julie Taymor where it proceeded to win numerous awards.

One of the award winning songs is *Hakuna Matata* with the meerkat Timor leading and the warthog Pumbaa playing a featured role as an ever-farting sidekick. Hukana matata is a Swahili phrase that means there is not a problem.

He found his aroma lacked a certain appeal
He could clear the savannah after every meal
I'm a sensitive soul
though I seem thick-skinned
And it hurt
that my friends never stood downwind
And oh, the shame,
He was ashamed
Thought of changin' my name,
What's in a name?
And I got downhearted,
How did ya feel?
Everytime that I... (farted, not said because of interruption below)

Hey! Pumbaa! Not in front of the kids!
Oh. Sorry!

Cartoonists

Cartoon art and illustrations making humorous or satirical reference to farting have been popular for many hundreds of years. They range from Edo Period Japanese woodcuts, to medieval lithographs at the time of Martin Luther in the 1500's, to political satire at the time of the American Revolution. Cartoon illustrations with or without humorous captions number in the thousands, and virtually all of them are readily accessible by a search engine on Internet.

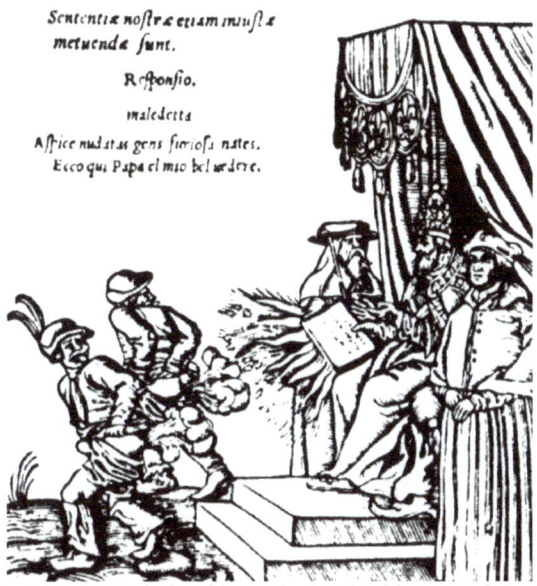

The Papal Belvedere by Lucas Cranach the Elder in the 1545 publication of Martin Luther's Depiction of the Papacy.

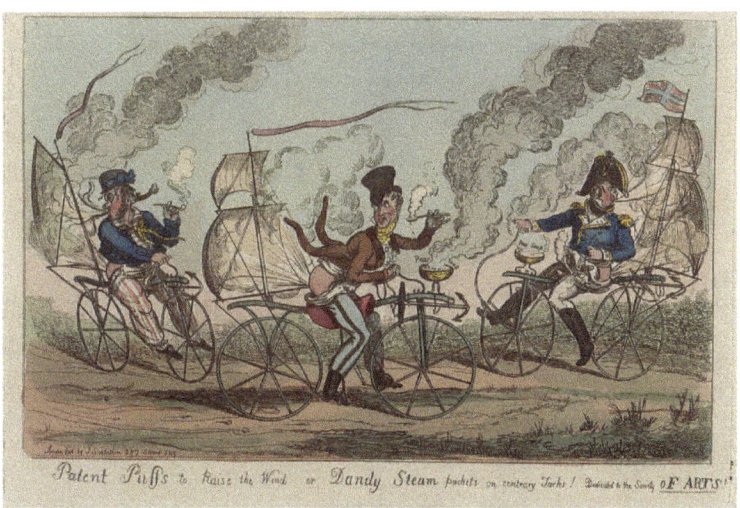

Patent puffs to raise the wind or Dandy steam packets on contrary Jacks! Dedicated to the Society of Arts! J. Sidebethem 1819

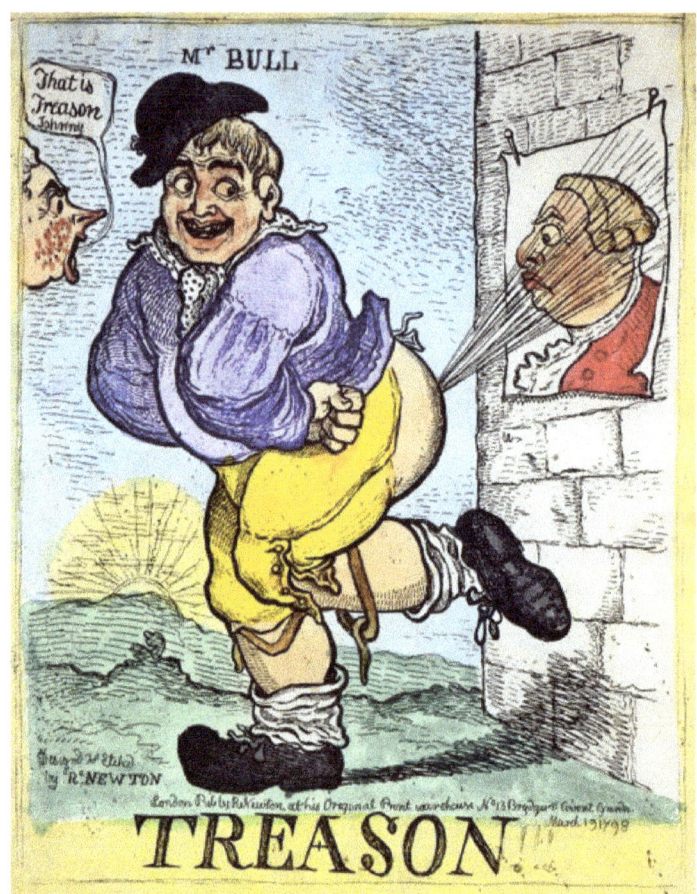
Richard Newton, Public Domain

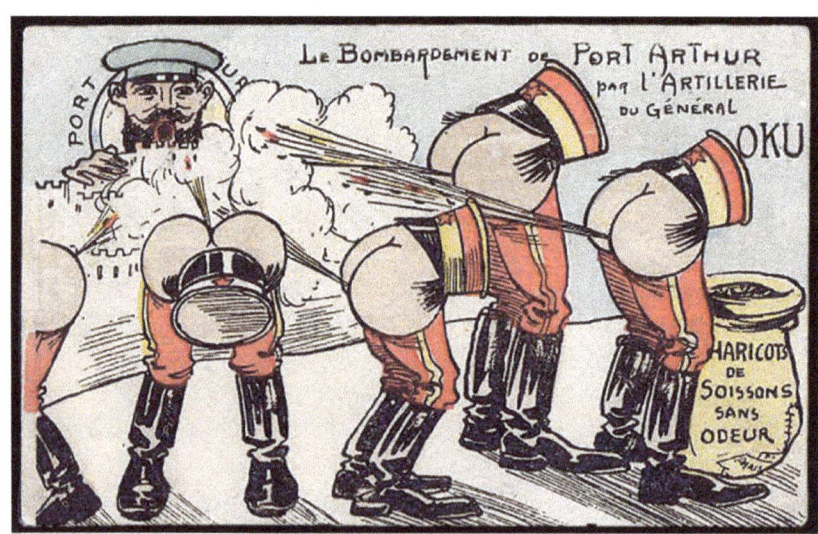

Artsy Fartsy: Cultural History of the Fart Volume One

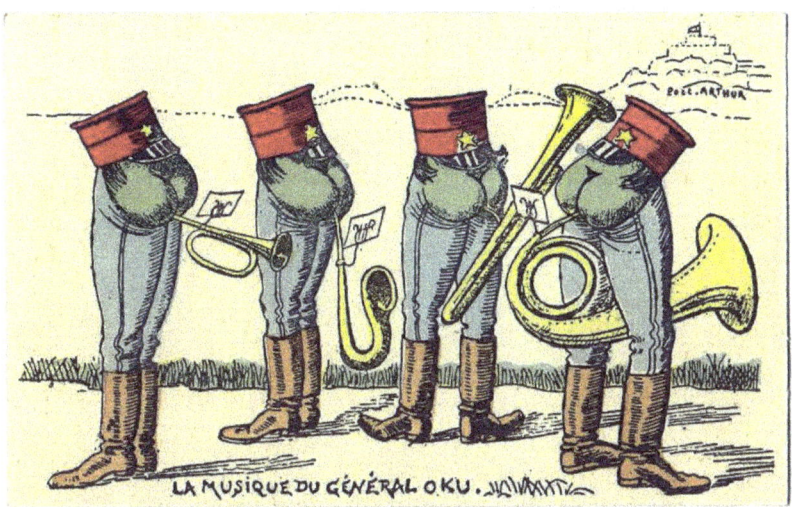

French cartoons from the World War One era. Public Domain

Children's Book Art

There has been a figurative explosion in the number of children's books on farts and other bodily functions. One of the early pioneering volumes was *Good Families Don't* by popular Canadian children book authors Robert Munsch and Alan Daniel. The clever, respectful, and witty volume was accepted for publication by Doubleday Canada but only on the condition that the word fart was dropped from the title.

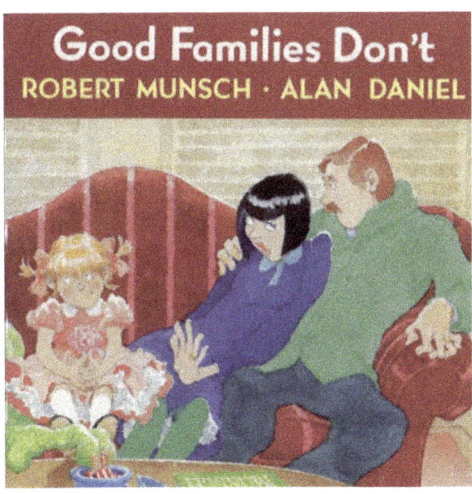

Since this occurred in the 1980's the word fart has reentered the mainstream vocabulary and entertaining and informative children's books with the word fart in the title have prominent window display. *The Gas We Pass: The Story of Farts* by Shinta Cho has become a children's bestseller.

Artsy Fartsy: Cultural History of the Fart Volume One

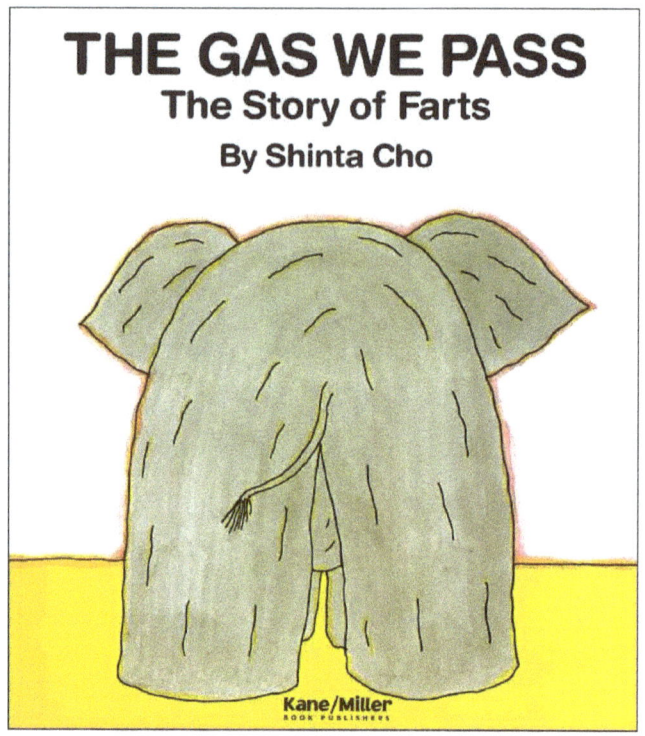

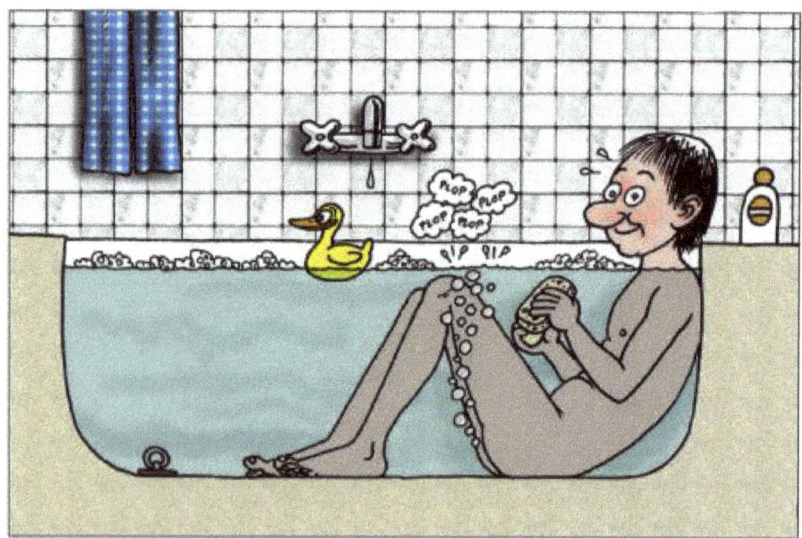

Illustration from the Big Bottom Book. www.toonpool.com/cartoons

Whimsical images of farts and farting are replete through the ever-growing library of children's books.

The Simpsons, Family Guy, South Park, Beavis & Butt-head

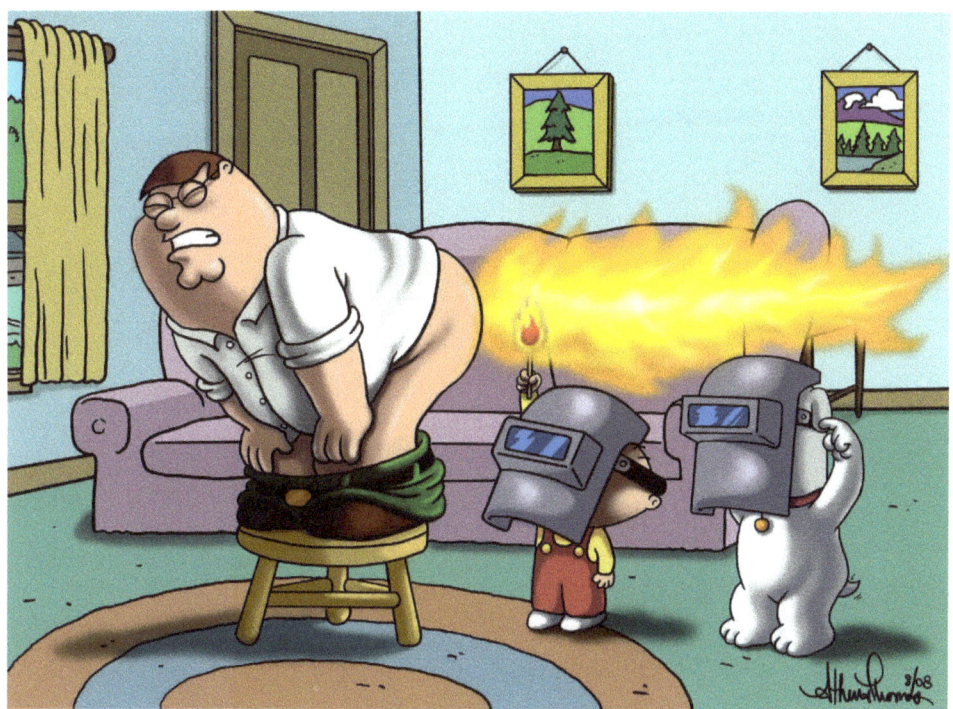

stuffpoint.com/family-guy/image

The satirical comedy cartoon programs Family Guy, South Park, Simpsons, Beavis & Butt-head, etcetera have become very popular and cult classics in the United States. Farts, bodily functions, sexual innuendo, and other subjects normally refrained from in television shows that may be watched by children are openly addressed. The levels of satire, sophistication, and comedy have encouraged a wide adult viewing population.

The Simpsons had an entire episode as a satire of the remarkable autobiographical story *The Diving Bell and the Butterfly: A Memoir of Life in Death* by Jean-Dominique Bauby. In real life the author had a tragic and severe stroke at the age of forty-four. He was able to communicate only through the blinking of his left eye. Using the painstakingly slow method of blinking code for each letter of the alphabet he was able to communicate with his family.

The richly detailed and moving account of his experience was transmitted letter-by-letter and published to wide acclaim. In the satire Homer Simpson is paralyzed by a spider bite, and his only means of communication is by farting, creating the sonic equivalent of Morse Code.

Chen Wenling

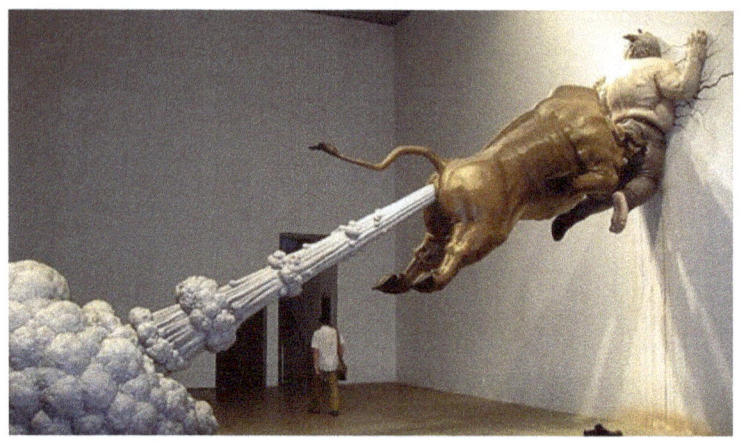

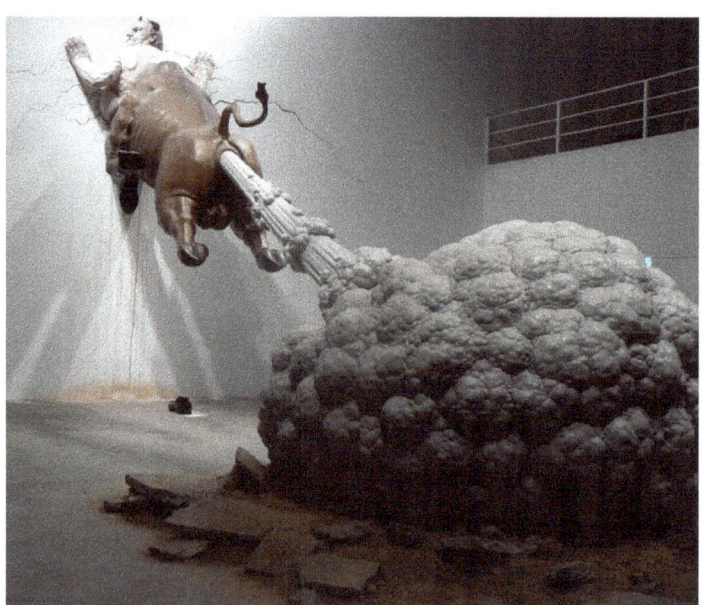

twitice.blogspot.com/2010/06/inspiring-bull-fart

Chen Wenling was born in 1969 in Anxi, Fujian China. He studied at the Xiamen Academy of Art and Design, and at the Central Academy of Fine Arts in Beijing. He is a contemporary Chinese artist now living and working in Xiamen and Beijing.

His highly distinctive massive sculptures are often described as raw, grotesque, or perverse. His thought provoking work is also seen as a compellingly fascinating commentary on modern society and has been exhibited in collections throughout the world.

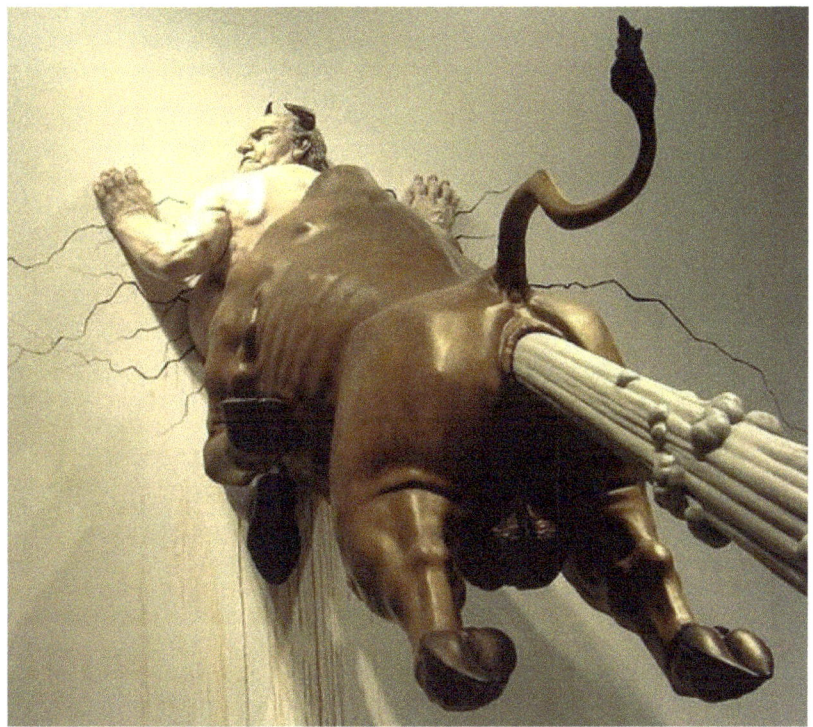

twitice.blogspot.com/2010/06/inspiring-bull-fart-sculpture

Ontario Ministry of Health

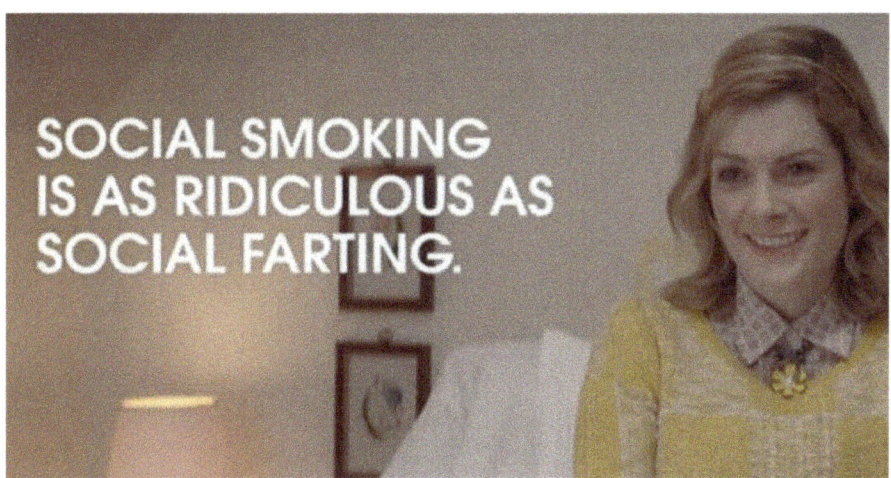

Ontario Ministry of Health video ad campaign against social smoking using farting as equivalent offense www.youtube.com/watch?v=w8762zEOkSo

Artsy Fartsy: Cultural History of the Fart Volume One

The Ontario Ministry of Health embarked on a public education campaign to curb tobacco usage. A common theme used by smokers to avoid the stigma of nicotine addiction was to describe their habit as a social smoker. The public education campaign focused on the denial as being analogous to describing oneself as a social farter than enjoyed farting while in the company of others.

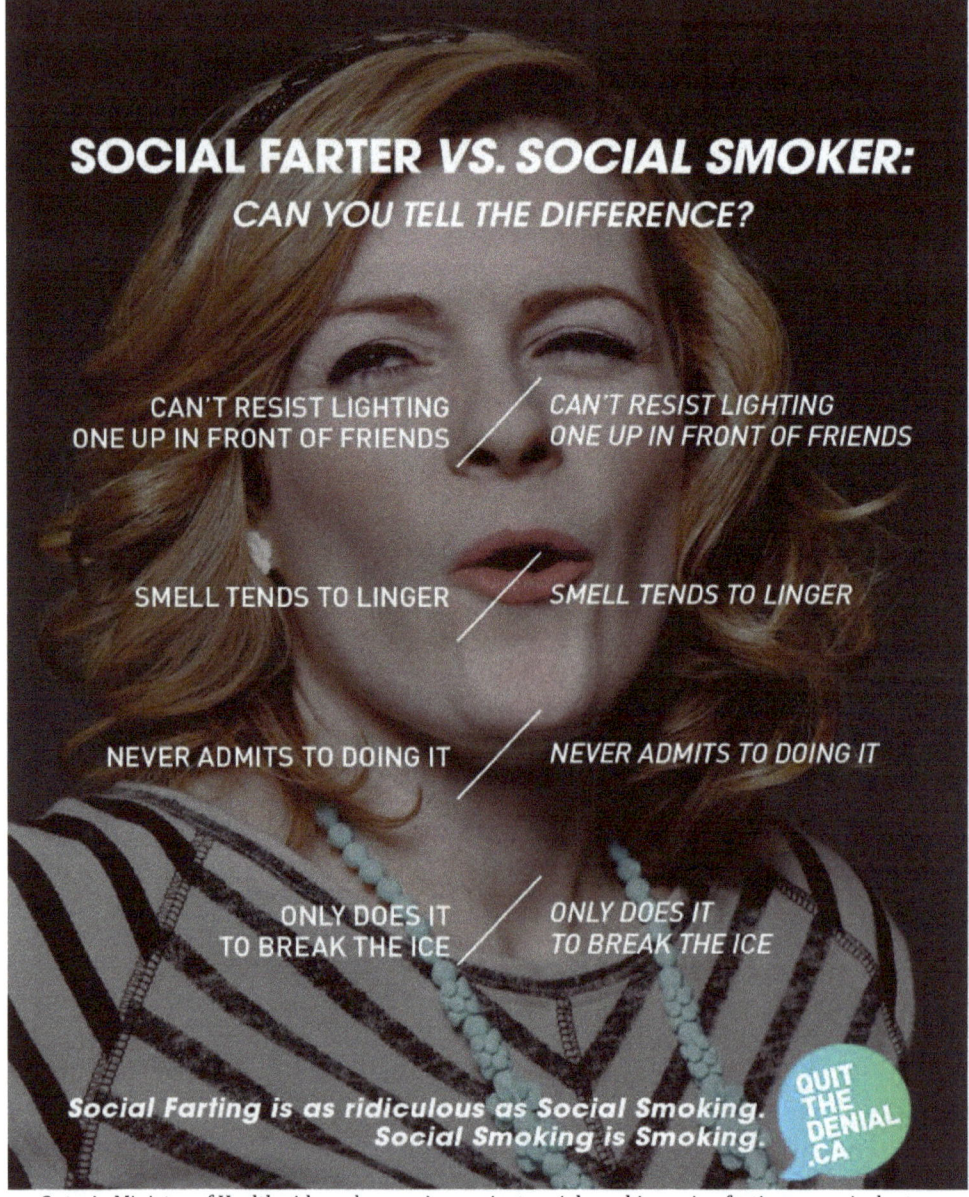

Ontario Ministry of Health video ad campaign against social smoking using farting as equivalent offense. Creative Commons License

Contemporary Advertising & Marketing

The media in Western cultures has seen rapid expansion of references to bodily functions and odors, especially the fart. The fart is now openly expressed in the content of cinema, television, radio, social media, Internet, etcetera. It is not surprising to see that the fart has become part of the content of marketers and advertisers, usually as a means of differentiating the products with an edgy youthful irreverence.

The Budweiser beer Super Bowl commercial referenced in a separate entry was a landmark public relations coup using the humor of a flammable horse fart. More direct references to farts has been employed in the advertising campaign of air-freshener company Poo-Pourri. Although the advertising campaign received a nomination as one of the worst ads by a national newspaper, it was a major hit on social media with over thirty million views. For a holiday themed advertisement Santa Claus is farting on the toilet while an attractive model sings a parody of a seasonal tune.

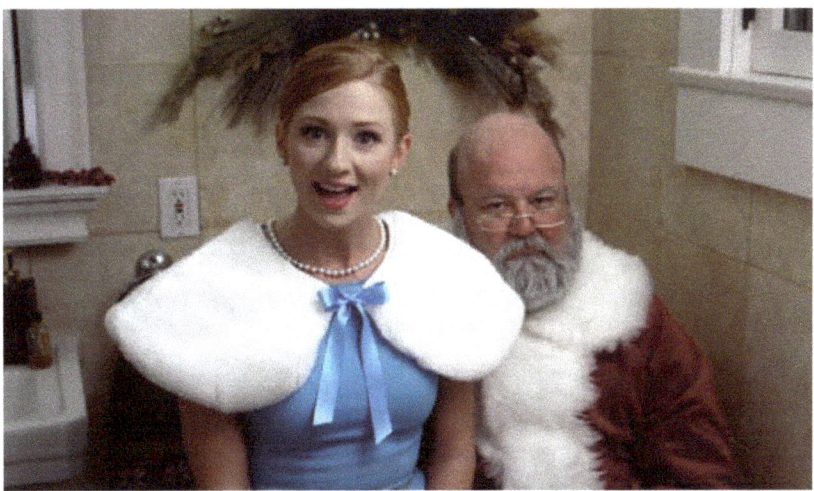
Poo-Pourri Advertising video www.ninjamarkweting.it

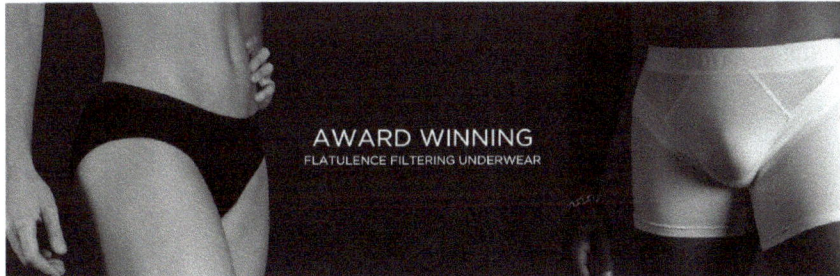
Shreddies advertising campaign for activated charcoal odor adsorbing underwear myshreddies.com

Artsy Fartsy: Cultural History of the Fart Volume One

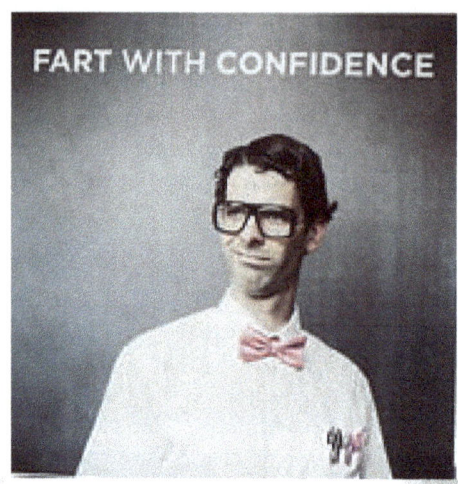

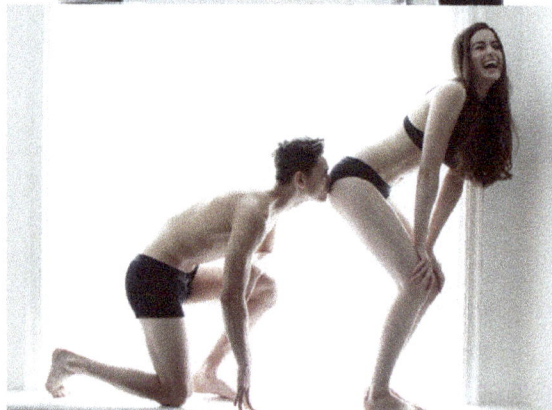

Shreddies advertising campaign for activated charcoal odor adsorbing underwear myshreddies.com

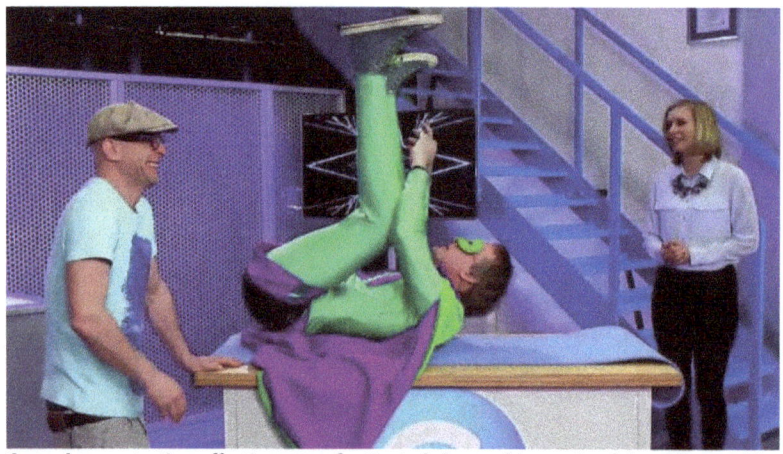

Mr. Methane demonstrating effectiveness of activated charcoal in a pair of shreddies on *The Gadget Show* myshreddies.com/media/?a=1

Artsy Fartsy: Cultural History of the Fart Volume One

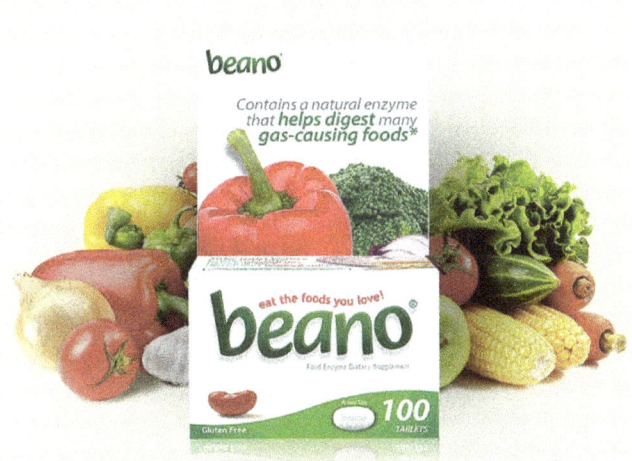

Beano was one of the first products to advertise a product designed to reduce intestinal gas. Its ad first appeared in Vegetarian Times

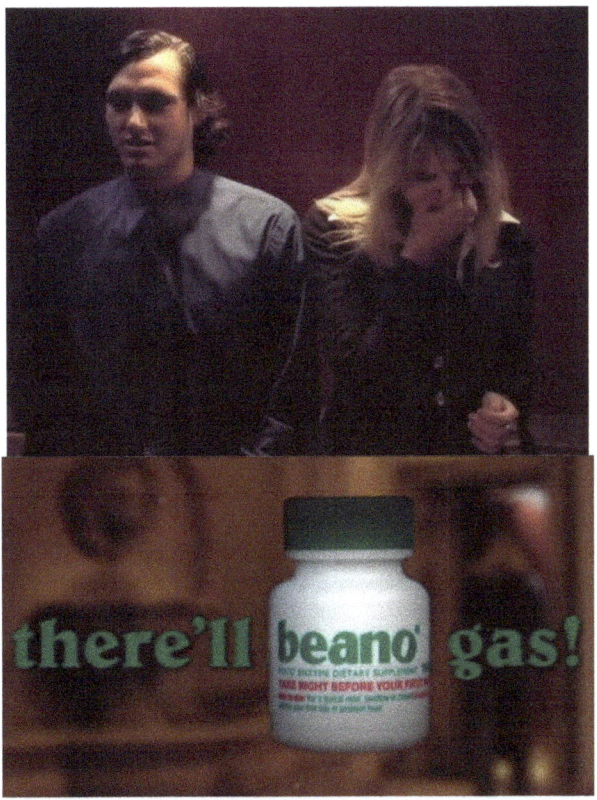

Beano advertised a humorous video of a person farting in an elevator ruining his chance encounter with an attractive woman. www.youtube.com/watch?v=sWkWdsx2ty0

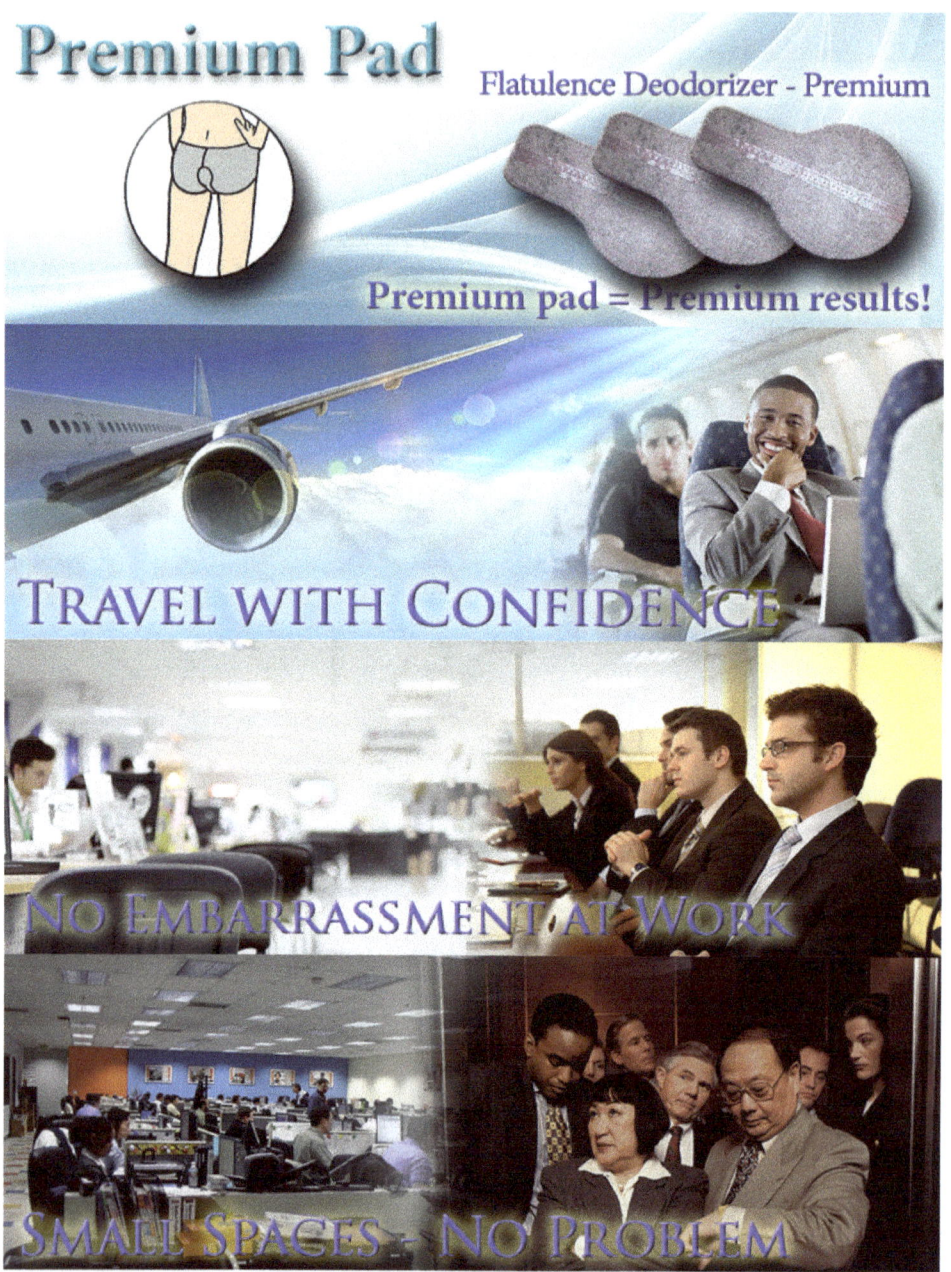

Flat-D advertises and markets a wide variety of activated charcoal products to adsorb the aroma of flatus and other body odors. www.flat-d.com

Artsy Fartsy: Cultural History of the Fart Volume One

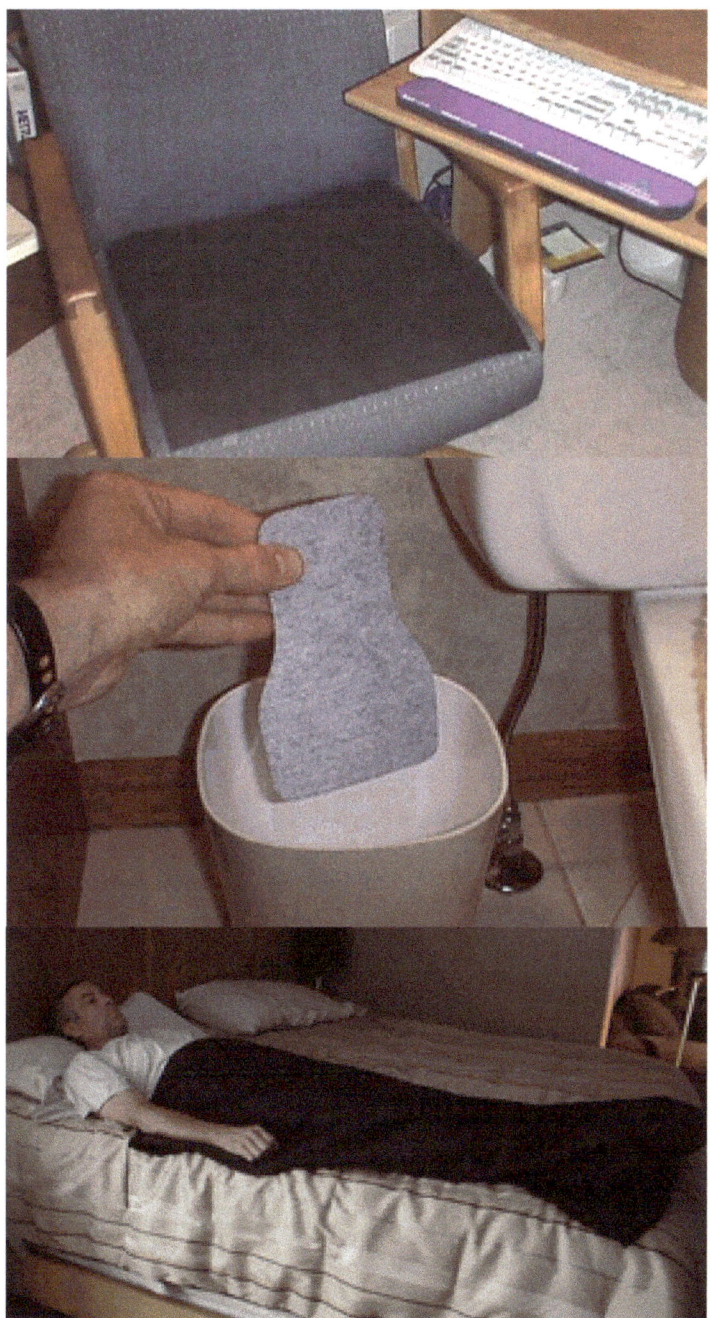

Flat-D advertises and markets a wide variety of activated charcoal products to adsorb the aroma of flatus and other body odors. Activated charcoal seat cushions, liners for underwear and clothing, and sleeping sack are amongst the numerous products they offer. www.flat-d.com/

Devrom is an over the counter preparation of bismuth subgallate and has been marketed for over fifty years as an internal deodorant. Bismuth does have antibacterial properties it may change the microbiome by reducing the organisms that contribute to offensive flatulence. Another bismuth product that has been popular in the marketplace is Pepto-Bismol, which is a bismuth subsalicylate. Bismuth subsalicylate is related to aspirin (salicylic acid) and does not appear to provide as significant relief from the unpleasant odors as has been reported with Devrom.

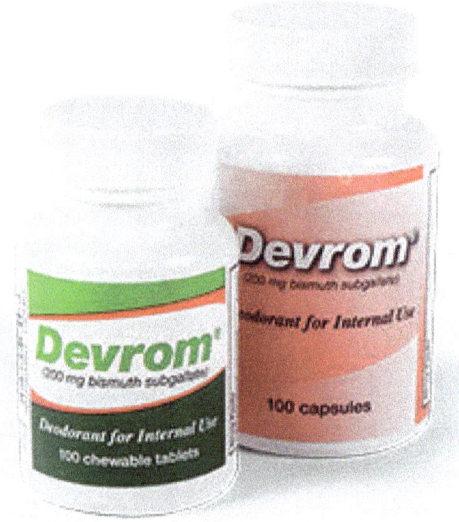

It has been particularly popular for individuals who have undergone gastric bypass surgery, inflammatory bowel disease, as well as those with ostomies, and others. With advances in surgery, and the ability to preserve sphincters or create artificial sphincters, ostomies are seen less frequently. This is where the intestinal discharge exits the body through an artificial opening, the ostomy, created at surgery. Because the bowel is diverted from the colon less moisture is absorbed and the feces may be semi-formed or liquid.

The more liquid form allows for the more rapid vaporization of volatile organic compounds and gasses that give rise to the feculent odor. In spite of being in otherwise excellent health, many individuals with these issues find themselves socially restricted in their activities because of concern about embarrassment or offending others. Safe and effective products are available, but many individuals are unaware and suffer unnecessarily because of the lack of information and understanding.

Over the counter anti-gas products often include simethicone a surfactant that reducers surface tension. Surface tension is the physical principle that underlies bubble formation. By reducing surface tension smaller bubbles coalesce into larger bubbles, presumably to ease the burp and belch to allow its release and to the relief of the relief to the gassy individual, not the one in their company.

Artsy Fartsy: Cultural History of the Fart Volume One

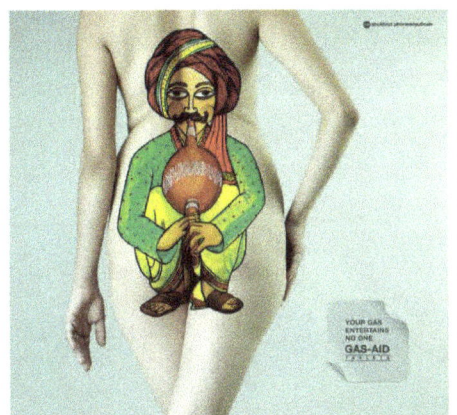
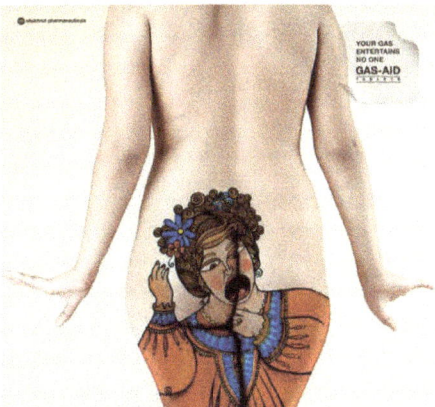
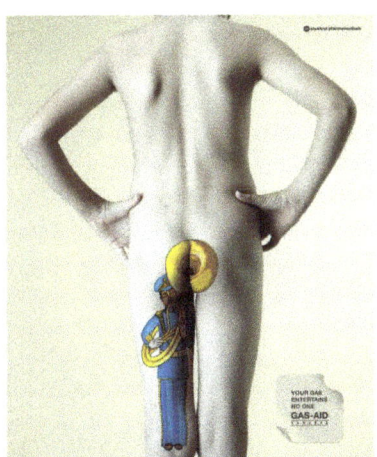
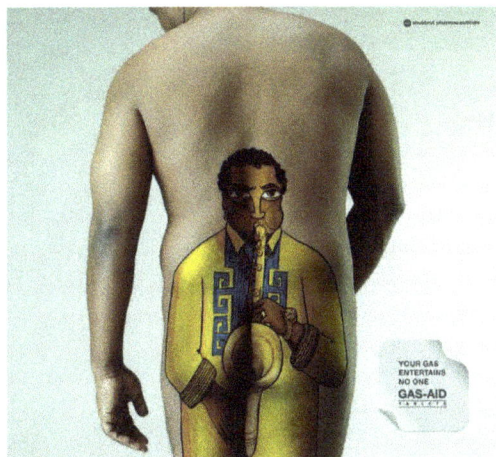
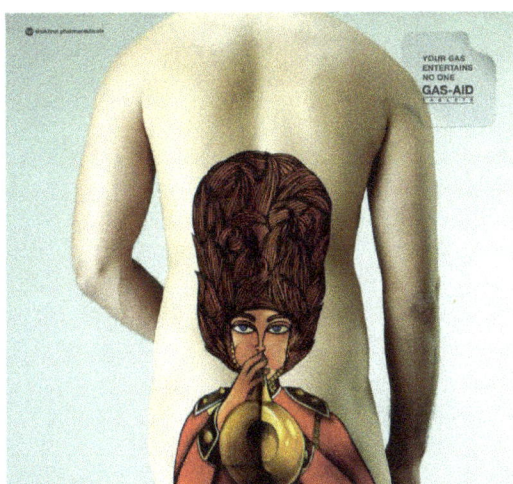

VII. Chronology of Fart in History

Bel-Phegor

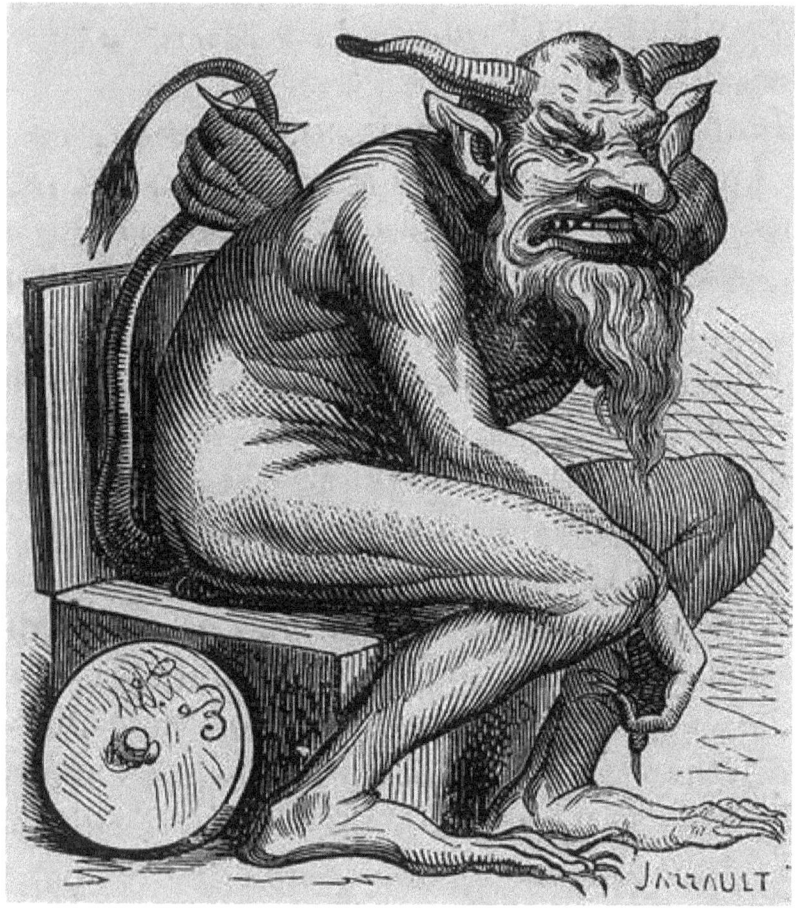

Illustration of Bel-Phegor(not in De Plancy's *Dictionnaire Infernal*, Public Domain

The ancient Pelusians of northern Egypt worshipped the god called Bel-Phegor with farts and bowel movements as religious offerings. More details of their practices are included in the work *Scatological Rites of All Nations* referenced under the entry for John Bourke. "The ancient Pelusiens, a people of lower Egypt, did (amongst other whimsical, chimerical objects of veneration and worship) venerate a Fart, which they worshipped under the symbol of a swelled paunch." — ("*A View of the Levant*," Charles Perry, M. D., sm. fob, London, 1743, p. 419.

Bel-Phegor is considered one of the seven princes of hell in demonology. He is thought to have been derived from the Assyrian Baal-Peor and was considered a god by the Moabites. He is referenced in John Milton's *Paradise Lost* and in Victor Hugo's *The Toilers of the Seas*.

Bible Prophets

The prophet Isaiah was believed to have lived around 700 BCE, and the prophet Jeremiah lived around 600 BCE.

Isaiah 16:11 Wherefore my bowels shall sound like a harp for Moab, and mine inward parts for Kirharesh.

Isaiah 63:15 Look down from heaven, and behold from the habitation of thy holiness and of thy glory: where is thy zeal and thy strength, the sounding of thy bowels and of thy mercies toward me? are they restrained?

Jeremiah 4:19 My bowels, my bowels! I am pained at my very heart; my heart maketh a noise in me; I cannot hold my peace, because thou hast heard, O my soul, the sound of the trumpet, the alarm of war.

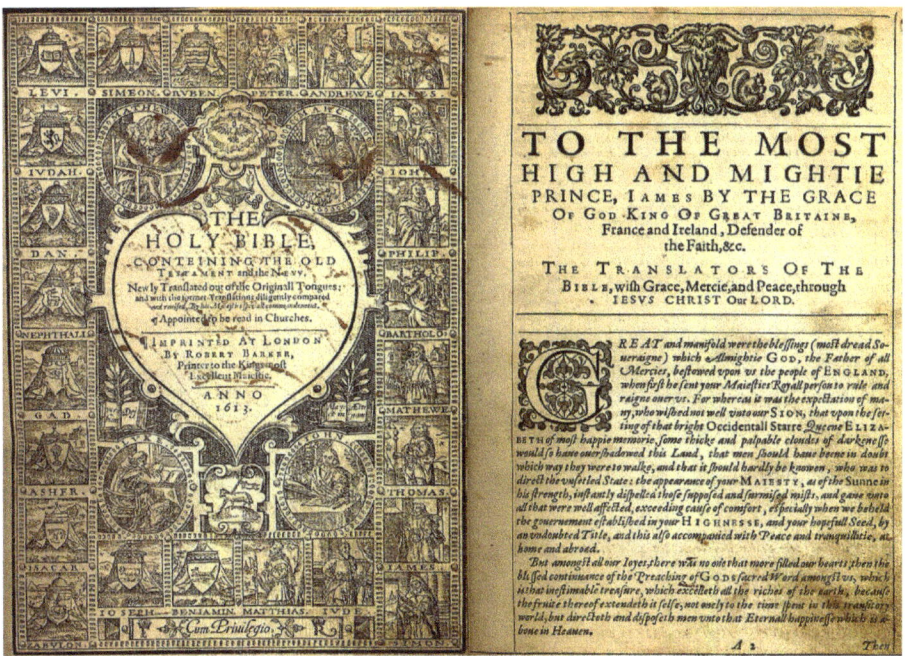

Frontispiece to the King James' Bible, 1611, shows the Twelve Apostles at the top. Moses and Aaron flank the central text. In the four corners sit Matthew, Mark, Luke, and John, authors of the four gospels, with their symbolic animals. At the top, over the Holy Spirit in a form of a dove, is the Tetragrammaton "יהוה" ("YHWH"). Public Domain

Pythagoras

Pythagoras of Samos (c.570 BCE - c.495 BCE) was a Greek philosopher from the region of Ionia, now found in present day Turkey. He was a pioneering mathematician, scientist, and the founder of Pythagoreanism, a mystic belief system.

The condition of favism has been known since antiquity and Pythagoras was a strict advocate of avoiding bean ingestion, perhaps due to the high incidence of favism in his area. Favism is a disorder where the sufferer is symptom free until forty days after the ingestion of fava beans. It is after this time period when acute kidney injury, hemolytic anemia, and other complications may arise.

Pythagoras and like-minded philosophers believed that beans and humans were physically and spiritually interrelated. Pythagoras also demanded that his adherents and students abstain from eating beans to avoid flatulence, as he believed that with every fart a small portion of the soul escaped.

He also believed that beans were the locus of the transmigration of souls and the belief directly contributed to his death. Chased by assassins he refused to take a path that would have allowed him to escape by going through a field, which contained beans. His philosophical belief in not harming beans in any way, even by walking through a bean field, resulted in his brutal murder at the hands of assailants.

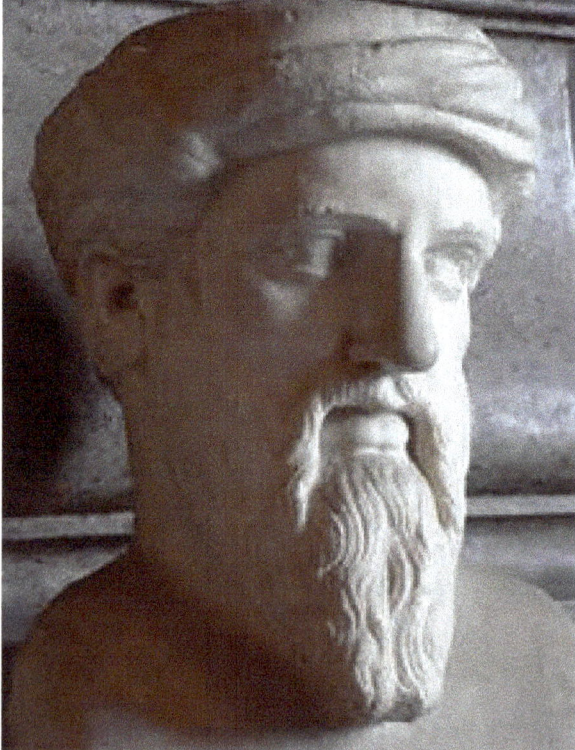

Pythagoras of Samos in the Capitoline Museums, Rome Roman Bust copy from Greek Original, Public Domain

Famous Quotations:

"Be silent or let thy words be worth more than silence."
"There is geometry in the humming of the strings. There is music in the spacing of the spheres. "
"Do not say a little in many words, but a great deal in few!"
"The oldest, shortest words— "yes" and "no"— are those which require the most thought."
"In anger we should refrain both from speech and action."
"No man is free who cannot control himself."
"Above all things, respect yourself."

Herodotus

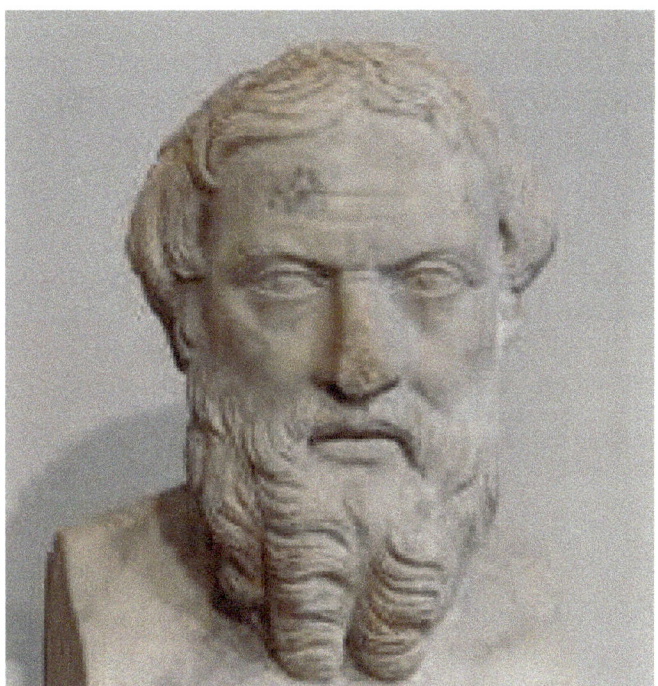

Head of Herodotus, Public Domain

Herodotus (c.484 BCE – c425 BCE) was an ancient Greek historian often called the Father of History for his classic volume *The Histories*. In the story of Apries below, a fart plays a role in starting a war that killed thousands and changed the course of history.

Herodotus on Apries:
Psammis reigned over Egypt for only six years; he invaded Ethiopia, and immediately thereafter died, and Apries the son of Psammis reigned in his place. He was more blessed than any former king, except the first founder of his family,

Artsy Fartsy: Cultural History of the Fart Volume One

Psammetichus I, during his rule of twenty-five years, during which he sent an army against Sidon and engaged the Tyrian4 at sea. But when it was fated that evil should overtake him, that which is alleged as the cause of it was something that I will say a little, and more about it in the Libyan part of this history.

Apries sent a great expedition against Cyrene, which suffered a great defeat. The Egyptians blamed him for this and rebelled against him; for they thought that Apries had knowingly sent his men to their doom, so that after their death his rule over the rest of the Egyptians would be strengthened. Bitterly angered by this, those who returned home and the friends of the slain rose against him.

Apries sent Amasis to dissuade them, when he heard of this. Amasis met the Egyptians and he exhorted them to desist; but as he spoke an Egyptian put a helmet on his head from behind, saying it was the token of royalty. This wasn't unwelcome to Amasis and for after being crowned king by the rebelling Egyptians he prepared to march against Apries. When Apries heard of it, he sent against Amasis Egyptian of good reputation named Patarbemis, one of his own court, with the order to bring Amasis live into his presence.

When Patarbemis came and summoned Amasis, Amasis, sitting on horseback, raised his leg and farted, telling the messenger to take that back to Apries. But when in spite of this Patarbemis insisted that Amasis obey the king's summons and go to him, Amasis answered that he had for some time been getting ready to do just that, and Apries would not find fault with him, for he would come himself and bring others with him.

Hearing this, Patarbemis could not be mistaken about his intentions; he saw his preparations and departed in a hurry, desiring quickly to make known to the king what was being done. When Apries saw him return without bringing Amasis, he didn't listen to what was being said and in his rage and fury had Patarbemis' ears and nose cut off. The rest of the Egyptians, who were still on his side, seeing this outrage done to the man who was most prominent among them, joined the revolt without delay and offered themselves to Amasis.

Hearing of this, too, Apries armed his mercenaries and marched against the Egyptians; he had a bodyguard of Carians and Ionians, numbering thirty thousand, and his royal palace was in the city of Sais, a great and worthy palace. Apries and his men marched against the Egyptians, and so did Amasis and his against the foreign mercenaries. So they both came to Momemphis and were going to make trial of one another in fight.

So when Apries leading his foreign mercenaries, and Amasis at the head of the army of Egyptians, in their approach to one another had reached the city of Momemphis, they engaged in battle: and although the foreign mercenaries fought well, yet being much inferior in number they were defeated because of this. But Apries is said to have supposed that not even a god would be able to cause him to lose his rule, so firmly did he think that it was established. In that battle then, as I said, he was defeated, was taken alive and taken to the city of Sais, which had once been his own dwelling but from then on was to be the palace of Amasis.

Famous Quotations:

"If a man insisted on always being serious, and never allowed himself a bit of fun and relaxation, he would go mad or become unstable without knowing it."
"Men trust their ears less than their eyes."

Hippocrates

Hippocrates (c. 460 BCE – c. 375 BCE) was a pioneering physician who lived during Greece's Classical period. He is widely recognized as the father of modern medicine. About sixty medical writings have survived that bear his name. He was revered for the high ethical standards he set for physicians, which are codified in the *Hippocratic Oath* still recited today by many physicians as they graduate from medical universities and school.

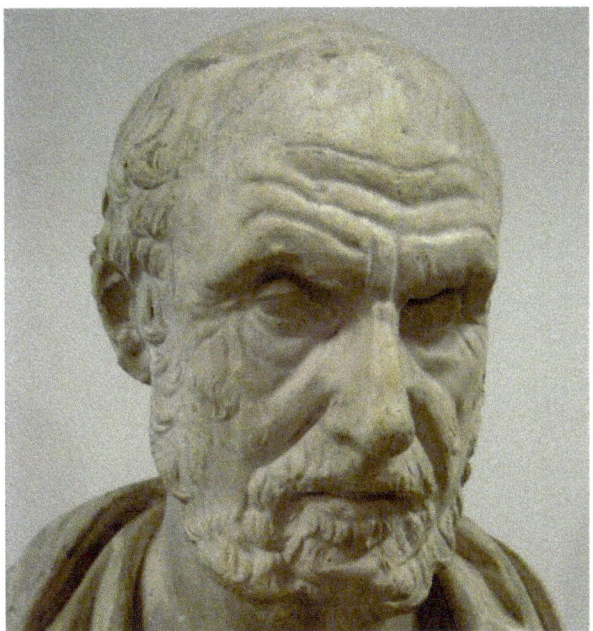
Hippocrates, Public Domain

As early as 420 B.C. Hippocrates had warned of the dangers of holding in a fart.

Treatise on the Flatuosities:

"It is better for it to pass with noise than to be intercepted and accumulated internally"

Famous Quotations:

"Let food be thy medicine and medicine be thy food."
"There are in fact two things, science and opinion; the former begets knowledge, the latter ignorance."
"Walking is man's best medicine. "
"It is far more important to know what person the disease has than what disease the person has."
"The natural healing force within each of us is the greatest force in getting well."
"All parts of the body which have a function, if used in moderation and exercised in labors in which each is accustomed, become thereby healthy, well developed and age more slowly, but if unused they become liable to disease, defective in growth and age quickly."
"The natural healing force within each of us is the greatest force in getting well."
"A wise man should consider that health is the greatest   of human blessings, and learn how by his own   thought to derive benefit from his illnesses."

Aristotle

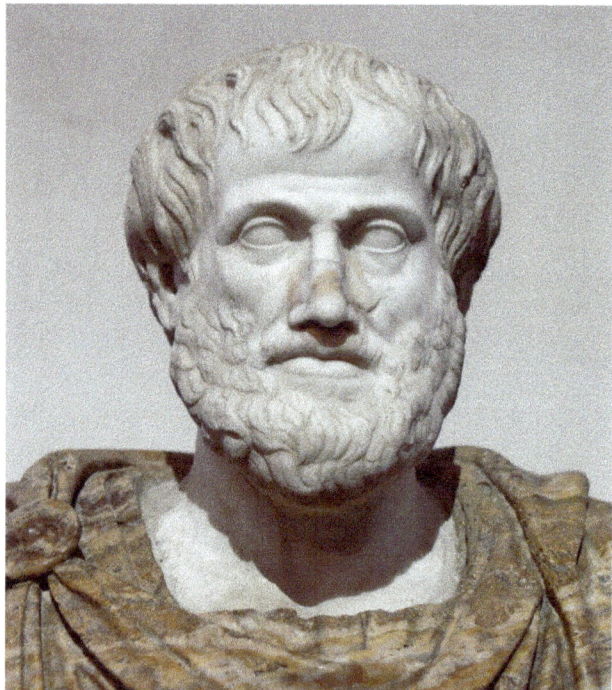

Aristotle, Public Domain

Aristotle (384 BC – 322 BCE) was a prominent Greek philosopher and polymath. He was a student of Plato, and the teacher and friend of Alexander the Great. Aristotle wrote on the digestive problems of elephants in his work *Historia Animalium*.

Historia Animalium:
Elephants suffer from flatulence, and when thus afflicted can void neither solid nor liquid residuum. If the elephant swallow earth-mould it suffers from relaxation; but if it go on taking it steadily, it will experience no harm. From time to time it takes to swallowing stones. It suffers also from diarrhea: in this case they administer draughts of lukewarm water or dip its fodder in honey, and either one or the other prescription will prove a costive.

The octopus ... seeks its prey by so changing its color as to render it like the color of the stones adjacent to it; it does so also when alarmed.

He also was a keen observer of other life forms, commenting on the color changing abilities of the octopus, both for camouflage and for signaling. His description of its reproductive process with the male sexual organ called the hectocotylus being detached from the male octopus and presented to the female with its spermatophores (packets of sperm) was not believed for over two thousand years, until his observations were verified by scientists in the nineteenth century.

Famous Quotations:

"Knowing yourself is the beginning of all wisdom."
"No great mind has ever existed without a touch of madness."
"Educating the mind without educating the heart is no education at all."
"Happiness is the meaning and the purpose of life, the whole aim and end of human existence."
"Anybody can become angry — that is easy, but to be angry with the right person and to the right degree and at the right time and for the right purpose, and in the right way — that is not within everybody's power and is not easy."
"Excellence is never an accident. It is always the result of high intention, sincere effort, and intelligent execution; it represents the wise choice of many alternatives - choice, not chance, determines your destiny."
"To avoid criticism say nothing, do nothing, be nothing."
"Patience is bitter, but its fruit is sweet."
"Those who educate children well are more to be honored than they who produce them; for these only gave them life, those the art of living well."
"He who has overcome his fears will truly be free."
"Those who know, do. Those that understand, teach."
"The antidote for fifty enemies is one friend."
"Pleasure in the job puts perfection in the work."
"It is not enough to win a war; it is more important to organize the peace."
"The high-minded man must care more for the truth than for what people think."
"I count him braver who overcomes his desires than him who conquers his enemies, for the hardest victory is over self."
"Hope is a waking dream."

Metaphysics:
"It is the mark of an educated mind to be able to entertain a thought without accepting it."

Metrocles

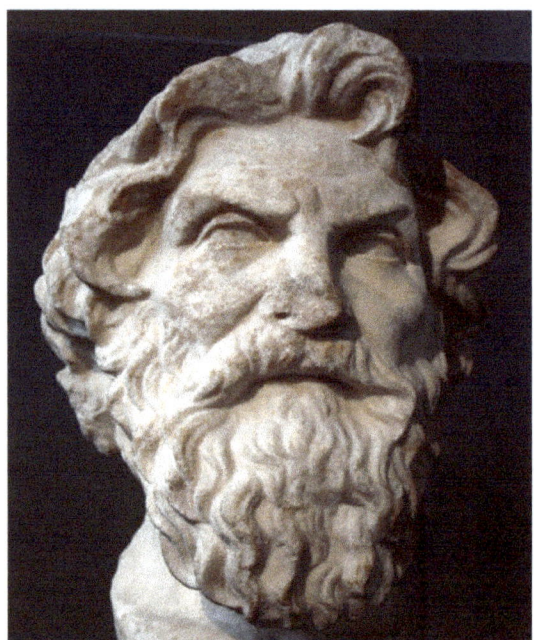

Metrocles, Public Domain

Metrocles (c.325 BCE), a philosopher who studied in Aristotle's Lyceum, accidentally farted in public while practicing a speech. He was so embarrassed that he attempted to commit suicide by starvation. Crates of Thebes, a proponent of a rival school of philosophy known as Cynisicm came to visit him and made a meal of lupin beans.

Crates farted and was able to convince Metrocles that farting was a natural occurrence and nothing to be ashamed of. Metrocles recognized that all of his education up to that point placed a higher value on social conventions and perceived good manners rather than true knowledge. From that time forward Metrocles was a pupil of Crates and an advocate of the Cynic philosophical approach.

Metrocles burned his own written work so very little of his writings have been passed down. What he is recognized for is the initiation of writing anecdotes and maxims, which became a popular means of expressing philosophical wisdom. He collected thousands of anecdotes of others under the title *Chreiai* (Greek: Χρεῖαι) that translates as *Maxims*.

Cicero

Marcus Tullius Cicero (106 BCE – 43 BCE) was a Roman philosopher, statesman, lawyer, and orator.

Cicero wrote: "The fart as well as the burp must be permitted".

Cicero's *Heuristics* starts with "Open with a fart joke, use Farticus if you don't have another."

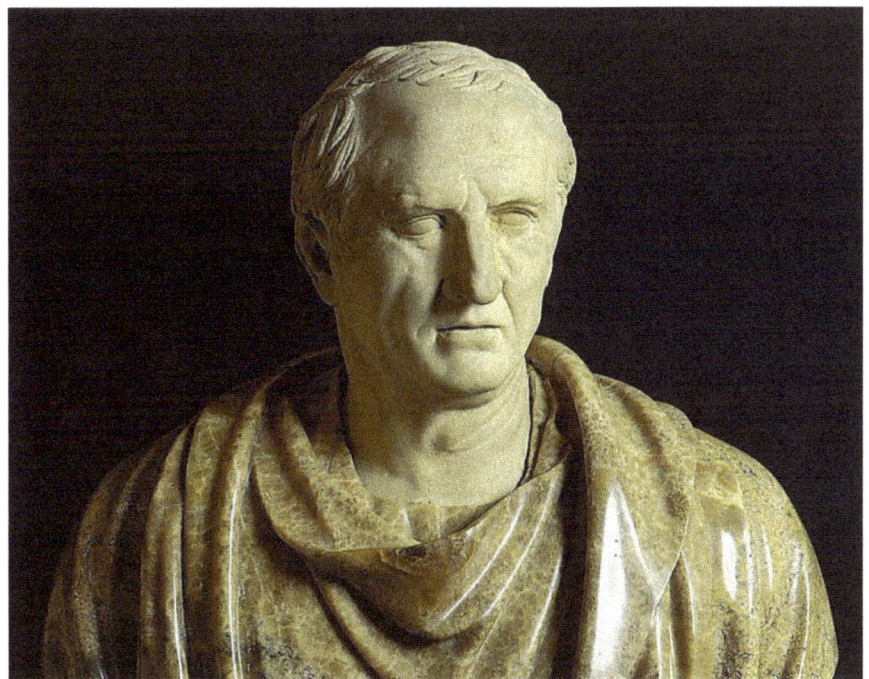
Cicero, Public Domain

Cicero's famous Farticus was possibly the world's first limerick.

There once was a man named Farticus
Who bravely fought beside Spartacus.
He let one rip,
His gladius slipped,
And we smelled no more of this Farticus.

Afflatus – Although it contains the word flatus, which is a commonly used as a synonym for fart, this word has nothing to do with a fart. Flatus is Latin for a blowing, breathing, or a wind. Afflatus is a word first used by Cicero in his volume *De Natura Deorum* (The Nature of the Gods). In his book it is used a phrase for a sudden rush of unexpected breath, a fresh inspiration. In fact the word inspiration is derived by inspire, to breath as well as to have a creative thought or new idea. Afflatus thus can mean a divine inspiration. The only way to associate it with a fart is to consider it to be the exact opposite of a brain fart (see separate entry under fart colloquialisms idioms).

Famous Quotations:

"Six mistakes mankind keeps making century after century:
Believing that personal gain is made by crushing others;
Worrying about things that cannot be changed or corrected;
Insisting that a thing is impossible because we cannot accomplish it;
Refusing to set aside trivial preferences;
Neglecting development and refinement of the mind;
Attempting to compel others to believe and live as we do."
"Friendship improves happiness, and abates misery, by doubling our joys, and dividing our grief"
"Gratitude is not only the greatest of virtues, but the parent of all others."
"For books are more than books, they are the life, the very heart and core of ages past, the reason why men worked and died, the essence and quintessence of their lives."
"If we are not ashamed to think it, we should not be ashamed to say it."
"Politicians are not born; they are excreted."
"Dum Spiro, spero- As long as I breathe, I hope."
"The life given us, by nature is short; but the memory of a well-spent life is eternal."

Claudius

Tiberius Claudius Caesar Augustus Germanicus (13 BCE – 54 AD) commonly known as Claudius became the fourth emperor of the Roman Empire upon the assassination his predecessor Caligula. Caligula was a flamboyant and notorious leader, and had made his horse a member of the Roman Senate amongst other actions, which raised questions of his sanity.

Claudius had numerous infirmities and was not considered either very intelligent or sophisticated but managed to be a fair ruler of the empire. He was reputed to be easily influenced by others, especially his succession of wives.

Tiberius Claudius was the fourth Caesar, the Emperor of the Roman Empire. Claudius had been made aware of an individual who had died as the result of a retained fart. To protect his citizens from a similar ill wind of fate he decreed that all citizens of Rome could fart at will in public or in private. There was no equal protection offered to the slaves. One can only wonder as to what their punishment might have been if they took the liberties of a citizen without permission, and farted in public.

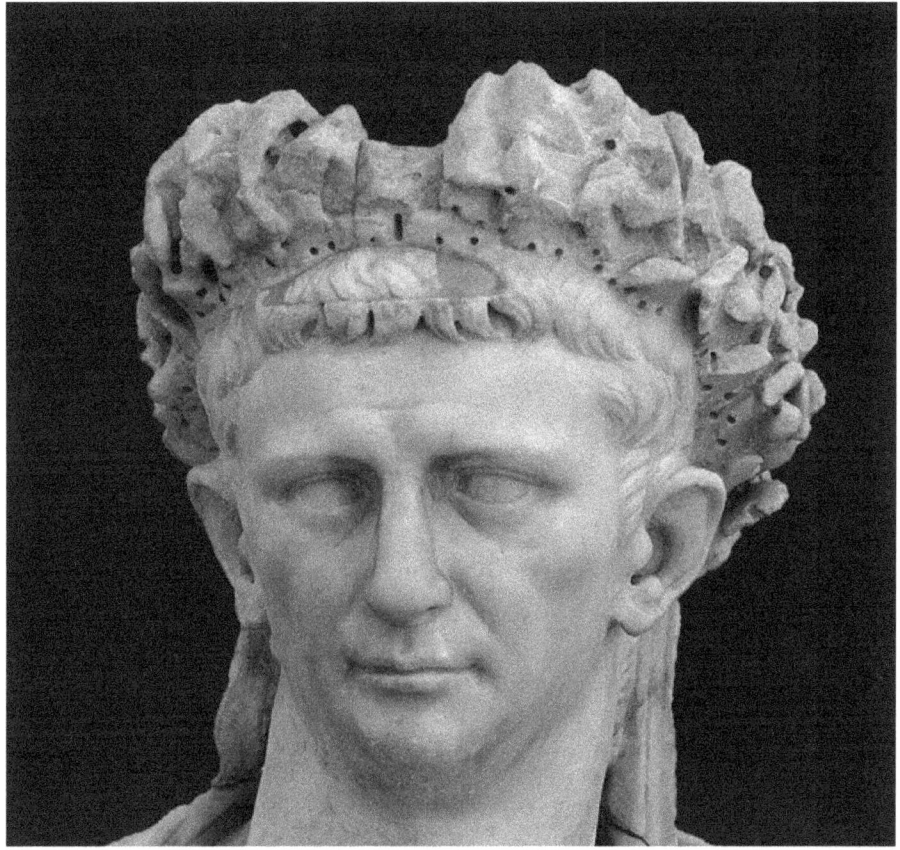

Tiberius Claudius Caesar, Public Domain

Famous Quotations:

"To do no evil is good, to intend none better."
"No one is free who does not lord over himself."
"No one is more miserable than the person who wills everything and can do nothing."
"Say not always what you know, but always know what you say."
"Acquaintance lessens fame."

Seneca

Lucius Annaeus Seneca (c. 4 BCE – AD 65) was a prominent Roman citizen, statesman, dramatist, Stoic philosopher, and humorist. He was a tutor and advisor to the notorious Roman emperor Nero, who forced him to commit suicide. Perhaps his suicide was preordained by his lack of reverence for previous Roman emperors.

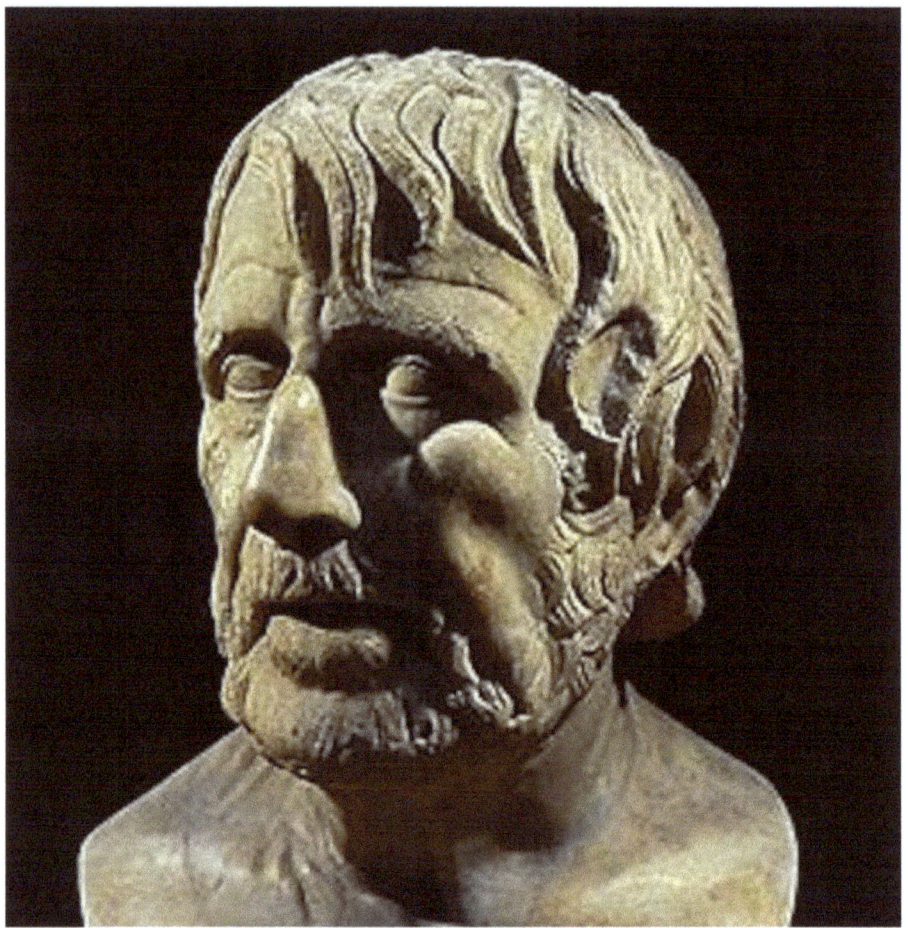
Seneca, Public Domain

In *Apocolocyntosis* or *The Pumpkinification of Claudius*, Seneca wrote of the late Roman emperor:

At once he bubbled up the ghost, and there was an end to that shadow of a life…The last words he was heard to speak in this world were these. When he had made a great noise with that end of him, which talked easiest, he cried out, "Oh dear, oh dear! I think I have made a mess of myself."

Famous Quotations:

"It is not the man who has too little, but the man who craves more, that is poor."
"Associate with people who are likely to improve you."
"Begin at once to live, and count each separate day as a separate life."
"As is a tale, so is life: not how long it is, but how good it is, is what matters."
A wise man is content with his lot, whatever it may be, without wishing for what

he has not."
"Luck is what happens when preparation meets opportunity."
"Religion is regarded by the common people as true, by the wise as false, and by rulers as useful."
"Religion is regarded by the common people as true, by the wise as false, and by rulers as useful."
"Difficulties strengthen the mind, as labor does the body."
"If a man knows not to which port he sails, no wind is favorable."
"Most powerful is he who has himself in his own power."
"True happiness is to enjoy the present, without anxious dependence upon the future, not to amuse ourselves with either hopes or fears but to rest satisfied with what we have, which is sufficient, for he that is so wants nothing. The greatest blessings of mankind are within us and within our reach. A wise man is content with his lot, whatever it may be, without wishing for what he has not."
"The sun also shines on the wicked."
"Only time can heal what reason cannot."
"Sometimes even to live is an act of courage."

Moral Essays, Vol 1
"Wealth is the slave of a wise man. The master of a fool"

On the Shortness of Life
"It is not that we have so little time but that we lose so much. ... The life we receive is not short but we make it so; we are not ill provided but use what we have wastefully."

Natural Questions:
"Timendi causa est nescire -
Ignorance is the cause of fear."

Natural Selections:
"The time will come when diligent research over long periods will bring to light things which now lie hidden. A single lifetime, even though entirely devoted to the sky, would not be enough for the investigation of so vast a subject... And so this knowledge will be unfolded only through long successive ages. There will come a time when our descendants will be amazed that we did not know things that are so plain to them... Many discoveries are reserved for ages still to come, when memory of us will have been effaced."

Flavius Josephus

Titus Flavius Josephus (c. 37 AD – c. 100 AD) was a famous Roman historian during the Jewish Wars and the reign of King Herod of Judea. In *The Jewish Wars* he describes a fart that led to the deaths of twenty thousand innocents. During religious festivals at the Second Temple of Judea built by King Herod, a contingent of Roman Guards was always present to preclude unrest.

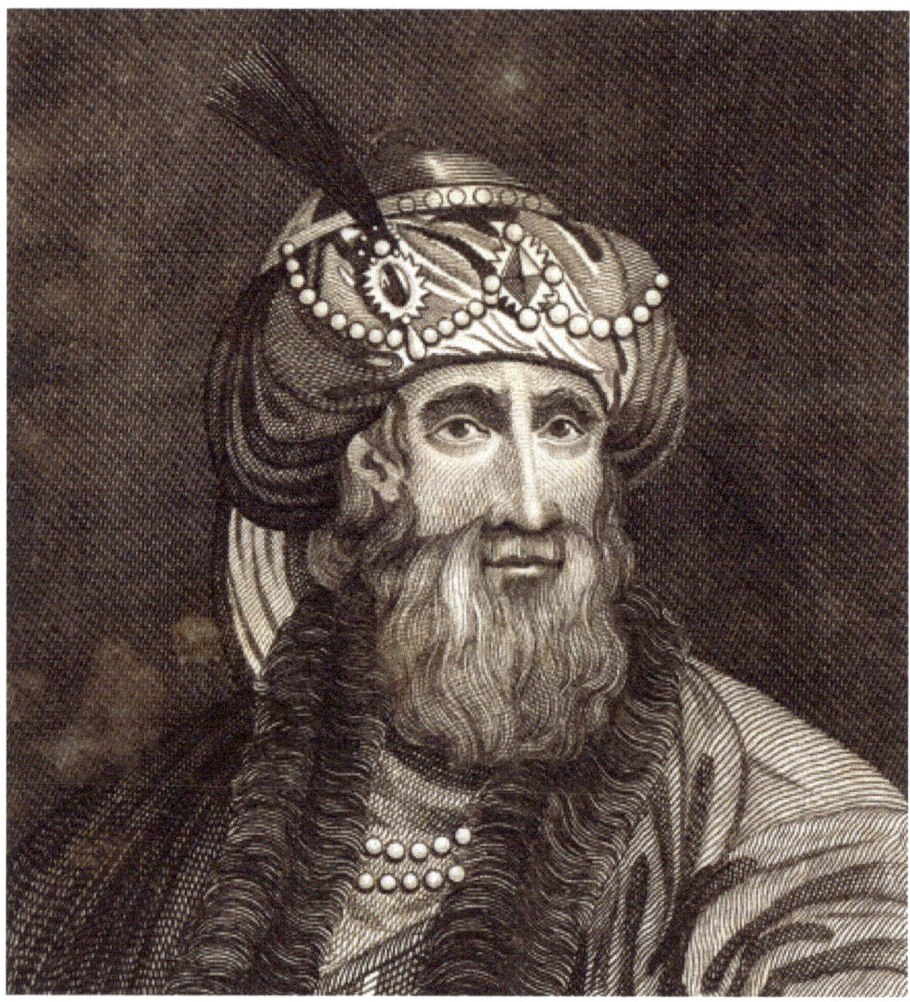
Flavius Josephus, Public Domain

One of the guards raised his garment, mooned the assembled worshippers and let loose a loud cannon blast of a fart. Outraged at the sacrilegious and offensive behavior they noisily demanded that the commander of the guards, Cumanus, punish the soldier.

Instead of punishing the soldier he rushed in additional reinforcements to prevent any further unrest and in doing so started a stampede of religious pilgrims for the exits. As Josephus describes the crush of people in the crowded temple plaza led to the deaths of over twenty thousand noncombatants trying to escape from a possible melee.

Plutarch

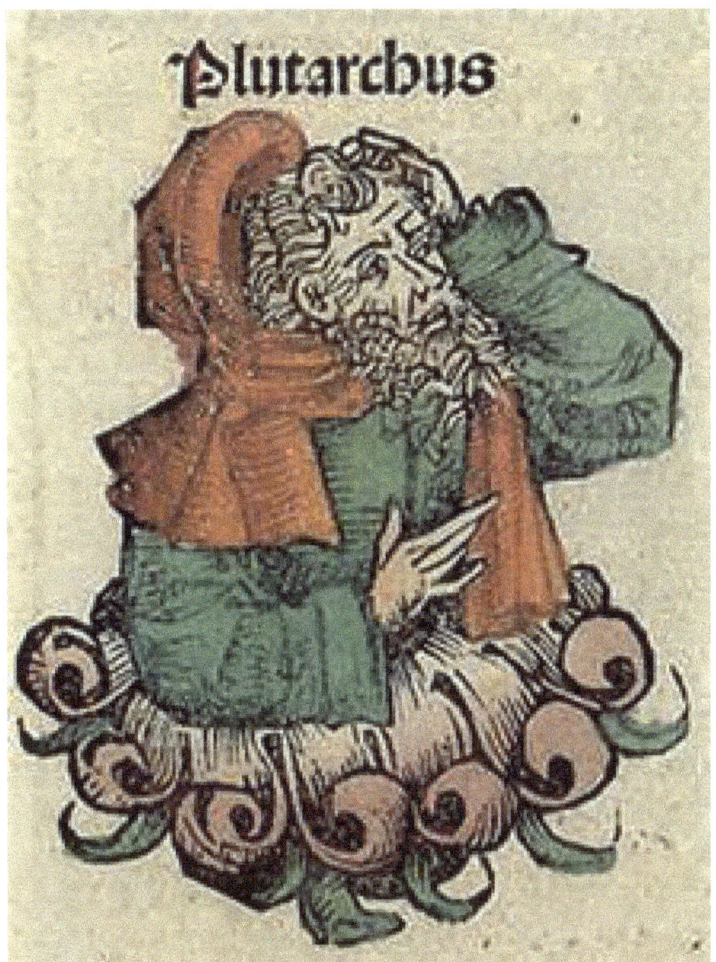

Plutarch, Public Domain

Lucius Mestrius Plutarchus (c. 46 – 120 AD) Greek historian, biographer, and essayist

Plutarch makes the following comments about pulse and beans.

"For the fruit, being new and flatulent, raises many disturbing vapors in the body; for it is not likely that only wine ferments, or new oil only makes a noise in the lamp, the heat agitating its vapor; but new corn and all sorts of fruit are plump and distended, till the unconcocted flatulent vapor is broke away. And that some sorts of food disturb dreams they said, was evident from beans and the polypus's head, from which those who would divine by their dreams are commanded to abstain."

Famous Quotations:

"I don't need a friend who changes when I change and who nods when I nod; my shadow does that much better."
"The mind is not a vessel to be filled, but a fire to be kindled."
"What we achieve inwardly will change outer reality."
"To find fault is easy; to do better may be difficult."
"To make no mistakes is not in the power of man; but from their errors and mistakes the wise and good learn wisdom for the future."
"Neither blame or praise yourself."
"Character is simply habit long continued."

Babylonian Talmud

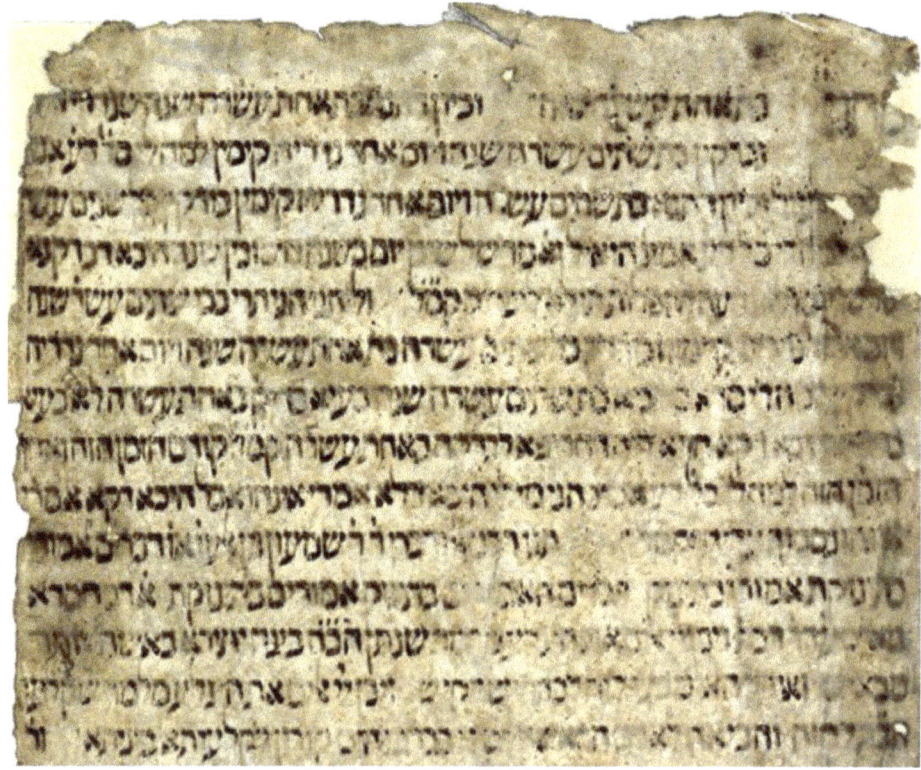

Babylonian Talmud Public Domain

It covers Judaic laws, ethics, philosophy, history, customs, controversy, heritage, and traditions amongst other subjects. It addresses the subject of flatus, and in deference to the holy scriptures of *The Torah* (Biblical Old Testament) it comments that it is forbidden to read or study *The Torah* in the presence of one's own flatus. It makes an exception for the flatus of others if it accidently passed in their sleep. It comments further on an exception to the exception, regarding the most sacred of prayers, known as *Shema Yisrael* (Hear O' Israel: The Lord our God, the Lord is One. Reciting the *Shema* prayer is forbidden in the presence of flatus, even that of others accidently passed. (*Babylonian Talmud*, Tractate Berachot 25a)

The Babylonian Talmud (Hebrew teach, study) is an extensive treatise and commentary on the central oral teachings of Judaism. It was written by leading rabbis around the year 200 AD, following the destruction of the second Jewish Temple and exile of the Jewish people to Babylonia. An earlier version known as *The Jerusalem Talmud* was written by resident scholars who remained in Jerusalem. *The Babylonian Talmud* is written in Aramaic and in the standard format is over 6,000 pages long.

Other Famous Quotes:

If I am not for myself, who will be for me? If I am not for others, who am I for? And if not now, when?
"The highest form of wisdom is kindness"
"Who is wise? One who learns from all."
"You can educate a fool, but you cannot make him think"
"To break an oral agreement which is not legally binding is morally wrong"
"A person will be called to account on Judgment Day for every permissible thing he might have enjoyed but did not."
"Whoever destroys a single life is as guilty as though he had destroyed the entire world; and whoever rescues a single life earns as much merit as though he had rescued the entire world"
"For the unlearned, old age is winter; for the learned it is the season of the harvest."
"No labor, however humble, is dishonoring."
"Who is rich? He that rejoices in his portion"
"Who can protest an injustice but does not is an accomplice to the act"
"This is the punishment of a liar: he is not believed, even when he speaks the truth."
"If silence be good for the wise, how much better for fools"
"More people die from over-eating than from undernourishment"
"Loving kindness is greater than laws; and the charities of life are more than all ceremonies."
"The end result of wisdom is... good deeds."
"There are stars who's light only reaches the earth long after they have fallen apart. There are people who's remembrance gives light in this world, long after they have passed away. This light shines in our darkest nights on the road we must follow."
"If one man says to thee, ''Thou art a donkey',' pay no heed. If two speak thus, purchase a saddle."

Elagabalus

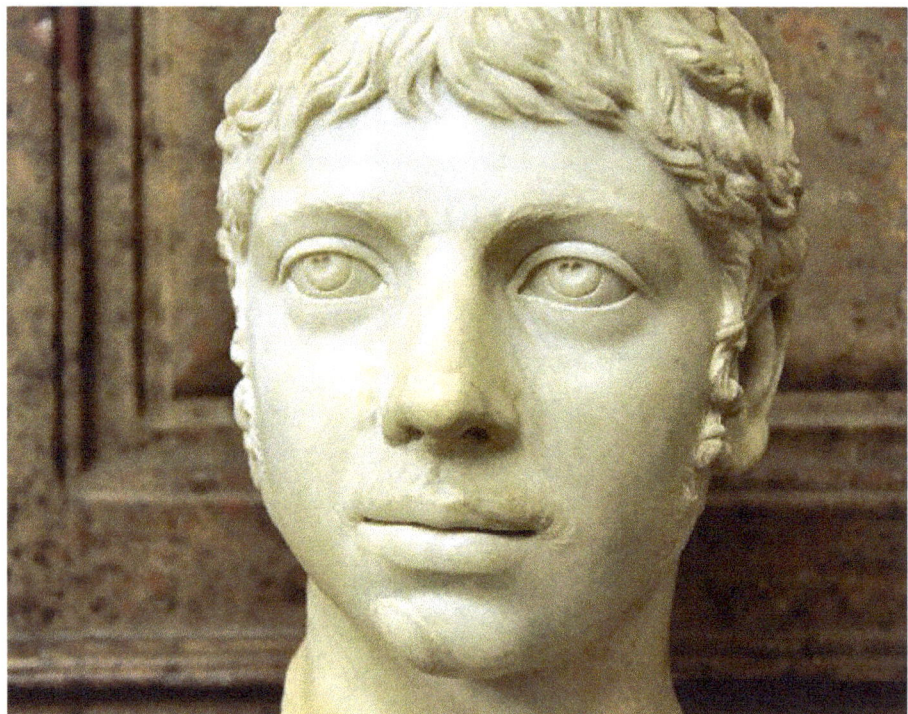
Elagabalus, Public Domain

Elagabalus, Marcus Aurelius Antoninus Augustus, (c. 203 AD – 222 AD) was Roman Emperor from 218 to 222. According to the findings of archeologist Warwick Ball the Roman Emperor Elagabalus played practical jokes on his guests. At dinner parties he would place whoopee cushion like devices under their seats from which fart like sounds would emanate.

He showed a disregard for Roman traditions and taboos, insulted the Roman Senate, the common people, and his own protectors the Praetorian Guard. It is therefore not terribly surprising that he was assassinated at age eighteen.

Whoopee Cushion

A whoopee cushion is a device used as a practical joke which mimics the sound of flatulence when compressed. It is commonly placed on a chair or cushion so that the sound is generated when someone sits on it. It is typically constructed as a rubber bladder, which is inflated with air.

A vibrating exit flap creates an audible fart like sound that is generated when sat upon. The modern commercially successful version was developed in the 1920s by the JEM Rubber Co. of Toronto, Canada. A more discrete alternate remote controlled version that can be hidden under a chair electronically generates prerecorded fart sounds

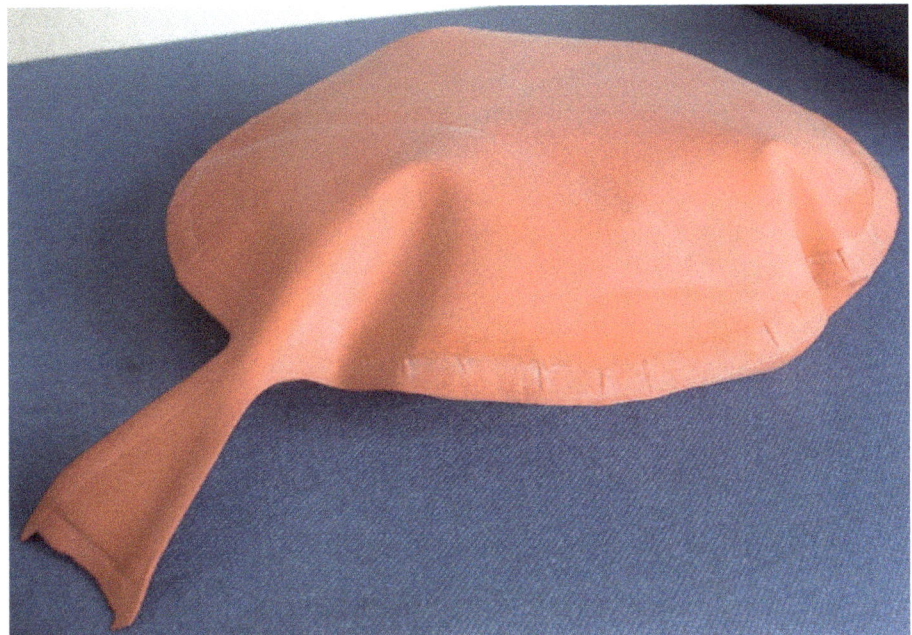

Whoopee cushion Creative Commons License

Yoga

Yoga is a physical, mental and spiritual practice that comprises many different schools and approaches. It has often been associated with the practice of Hinduism, Buddhism, Jainism and other belief systems that originated in the East.

The origins of yoga are not clearly defined but were thought to arise in pre-Vedic Indian traditions. The first documents ascribed to yoga are found in the Buddhist *Nikayas* and the *Yoga Sutras of Patanjali* recorded around 400 AD.
Yoga originally had been a religious practice and over thousands of years have become incorporated into secular wellness programs as well. Its effect on natural bodily functions, including intestinal gas were well recognized even in ancient times. Yogic masters and Brahmins in India practiced goze (flatus, eructation, belch) as a means of concentration in ridding the flesh of all-evil.

Yoga may provide benefit for some individuals with irritable bowel syndrome, especially poses that exercise the lower abdomen. It may also stimulate the passage of intestinal gas. In fact there are specific yoga postures designed to aid in the release of intestinal gas. It is not unusual for participants in a yoga class to experience the auditory or olfactory consequences of a fart. Perhaps it was the result of the successful assumption of the yoga gas release pose.

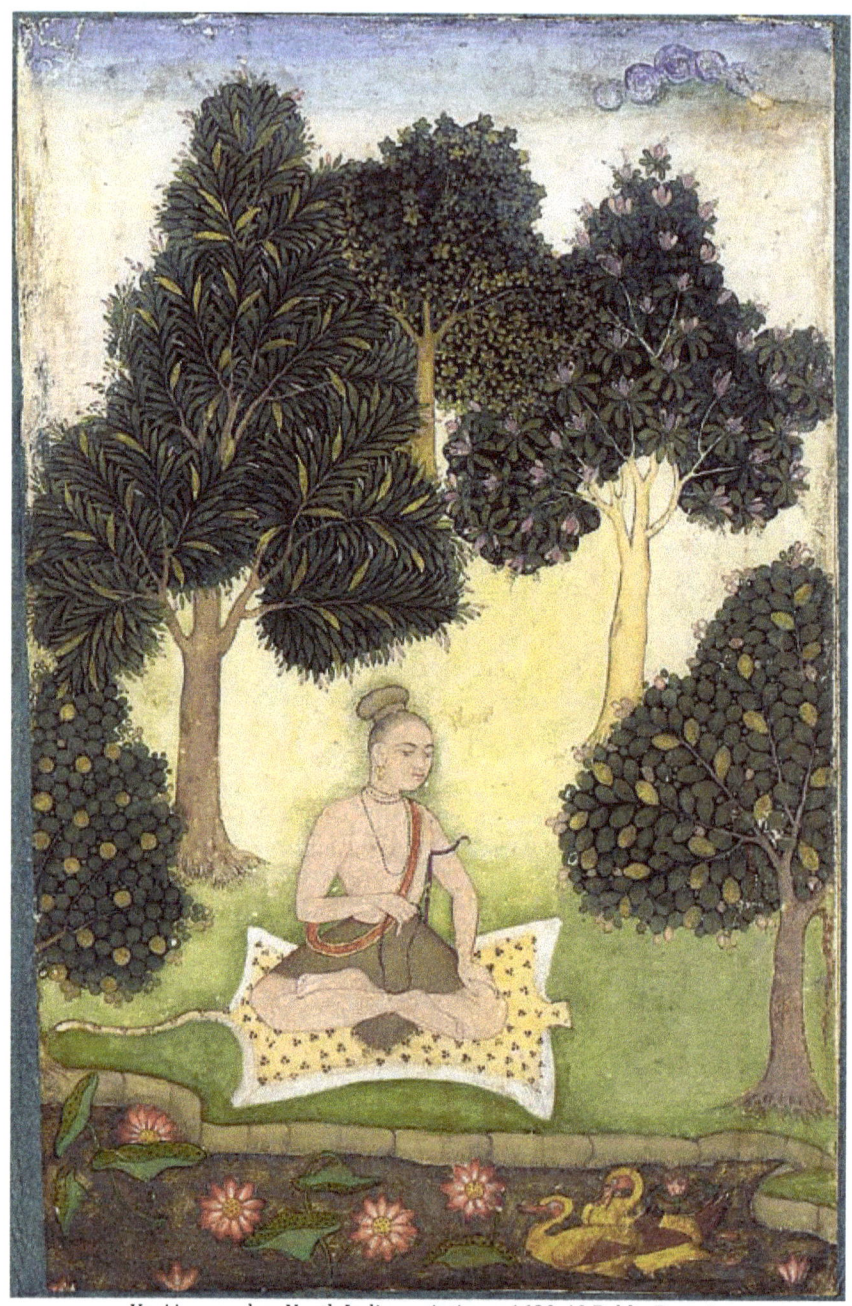
Yogi in a garden, North Indian painting, c.1620-40 Public Domain

Yoga is believed to help achieve the suppression of consciousness and the reaching towards enlightenment through union with the Supreme Being

(Nirvana). Among certain Brahmins, a spiritual blessing was required after each bite of food: He takes a little rice soaked in melted butter and puts it into his mouth, saying: "Glory to the wind which dwells in the chest!'

At the second mouthful, "Glory to the wind which dwells in the face!" At the third, "Glory to the wind which dwells in the throat!" At the fourth, "Glory to the wind which dwells in the whole body!" At the fifth, "Glory to those noisy ebullitions which escape above and below!" (Allen Edwardes: *The Jewel in the Lotus*).

Any general physical activity is beneficial as it increases bowel motility, yet there are a number of yoga postures that may provide additional benefit from compression and release of intra-abdominal pressure.

The Wind-Relieving Pose (Pavanamuktasana) is particularly effective. (Sanskrit: Pavana wind, mukta relieve, Asana Posture)

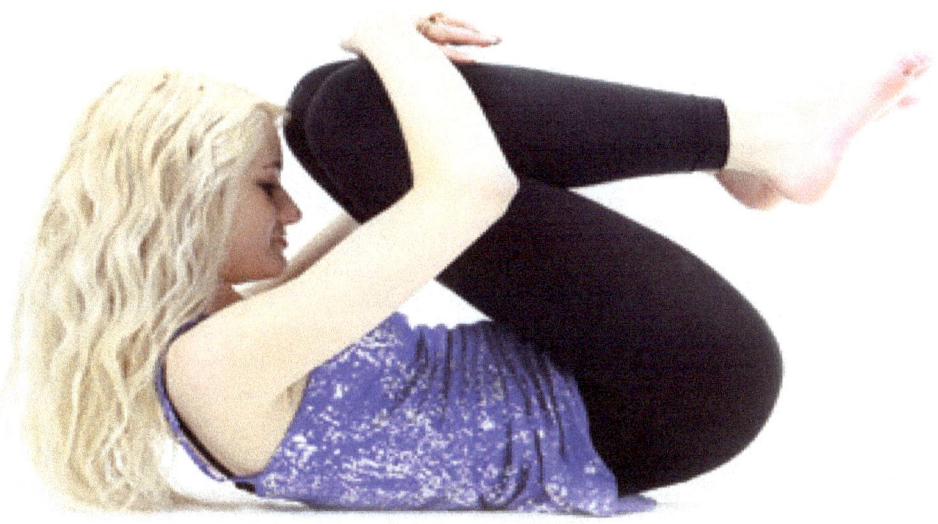

Pavanamuktasana (wind releasing yoga pose) www.a2zyoga.com Creative Commons License

Technique:
Lie on your back, arms by your side and feet together. Inhale and as you exhale bend your right knee and flex your right leg bringing the right thigh up pressing on the abdomen.

Inhale again and as you exhale lift your head and chest up off the floor and touch your chin to your right knee. Hold this position for several more cycles of inspiration and expiration. Then relax and after a rest repeat the sets with the opposite side. After a second period of rest and relaxation repeat the exercises using both legs at the same time.

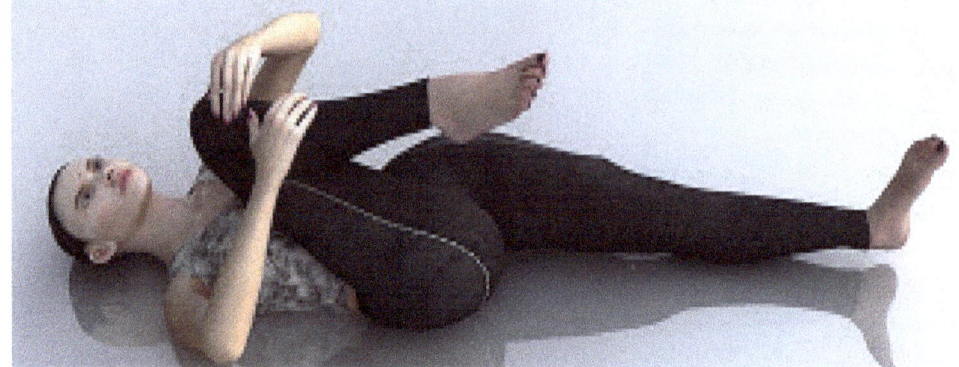

Pavanamuktasana (wind releasing yoga posture) alternative position
Technique: www.yoga-works.blogspot.com Creative Commons License

Avoid practicing the Wind-Relieving Pose (Pavanamuktasana) if you have high blood pressure, heart problems, excess acidity reflux or GERD, hernia, slip disc, neck or back problems, or are pregnant or if you feel any ill effects from the exercise.

Recognizing its role in general health and wellness it is no longer an exclusive religious practice but has become increasingly adopted into the mainstream. Of course any general physical activity is beneficial as it increases bowel motility, yet there are a number of specific yoga postures that may provide additional benefit from compression and release of intra-abdominal pressure.

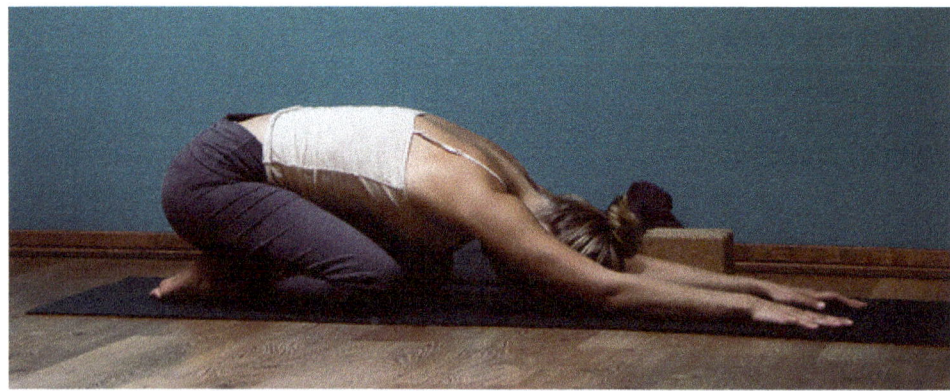

Balsana yoga posture flickr.com Creative Commons License

Sthala Basti, also called Vata Basti, Air Basti, Air Enema, is an advanced Hatha yoga technique that is best learned from an expert teacher. There are a number of different approaches and techniques but mastery of anal sphincter is a challenging practice. Once you master this technique you may not become as famous as Le Pétomane of the Moulin Rouge but you will certainly be able to entertain your soon to be former friends.

Sthala Basti starting from Paschimottanasana:
Sit with your legs stretched out in front of you and then bend forward halfway. You do not however fully place your upper body on your legs but only bend forward halfway. Perform Uddiyana Bandha by exhaling completely then taking a false inhalation while holding the breath. This flattens and pulls in the abdomen under the rib cage as if the chest was suctioning it.

The process is repeated many times followed by relaxation of the anal sphincter muscles to allow air to be drawn in with the uddiyanna Bandha maneuver. The air suctioned in is released as flatus.

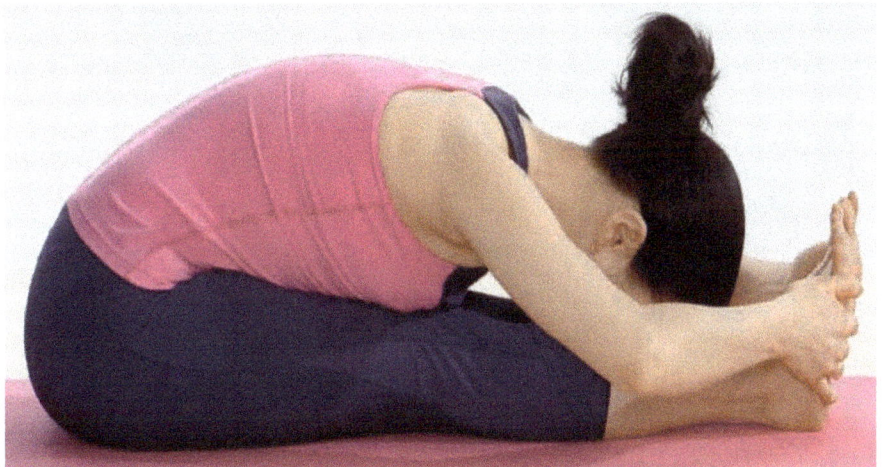

Paschimottanasana yoga posture www.yoganga.com Creative Commons License

Sthala Basti in lying Position

Lying on the back bend the knees up towards the chest and raise the buttocks. Practice developing control of the anal sphincter muscles by contraction and relaxation of the sphincter. When the sphincter is relaxed air suctioned into the colon is released as a fart.

Sthala Basti in Utkatasana

Sit in Utkatasana, also called the chair or lightening bolt pose, by squatting while standing with the knees bent ninety degrees backwards to thighs. The back and upright arms form a forward facing ninety-degree angle from the thighs. If necessary, until sphincter control is mastered, a hollow tube like bamboo or a catheter is placed in the anus and Uddiyama Bandha is performed. Air is sucked into the colon and released as a fart.

Other Yoga positions and moves that may be helpful include Balasana (Child's Pose) supported, Paschimottanasana (Seated Forward Bend), Supta Baddha Konasana (Reclining Bound Angle Pose) supported, Janu Sirsasana (Head of the

Knee Pose) supported, and Jathara Parivartanasana (Revolved Abdomen Pose).

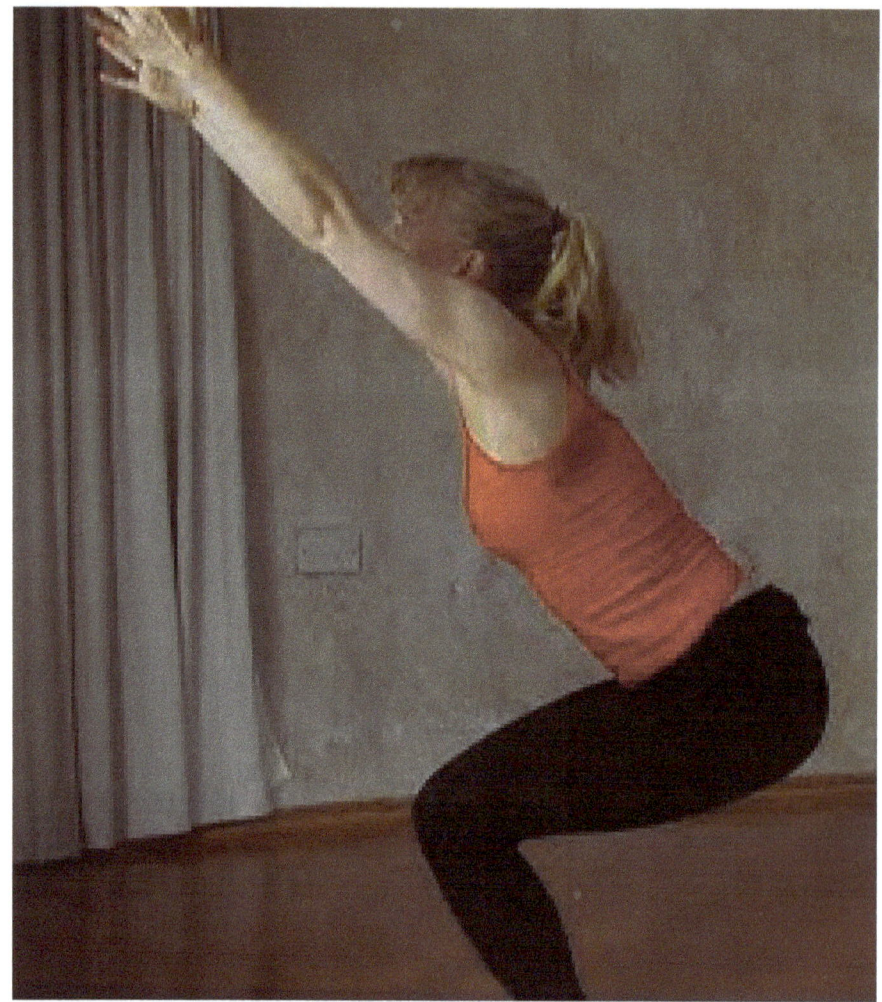

Utkatasana digplanet.com Creative Commons License

St. Jerome

Saint Jerome (Latin: Eusebius Sophronius Hieronymus (c. 347 AD – 420 AD) church scholar, historian, translator, and prolific writer. He was the single most influential person promoting the concept of celibacy for priests and nuns.

Much like religious figures of our day, who are most insistent on maintaining the high moral standards of others, he was implicated in a romantic scandal with a wealthy widow who provided funding for his monasteries. The writings of St. Jerome in a Letter to Furia 394 CE include the following admonition:

Artsy Fartsy: Cultural History of the Fart Volume One

It is good neither to eat flesh nor to drink wine – but with beans also anything that creates wind or lies heavy on the stomach should be rejected. I think that nothing so inflames the body and titillates the genitals as undigested food.

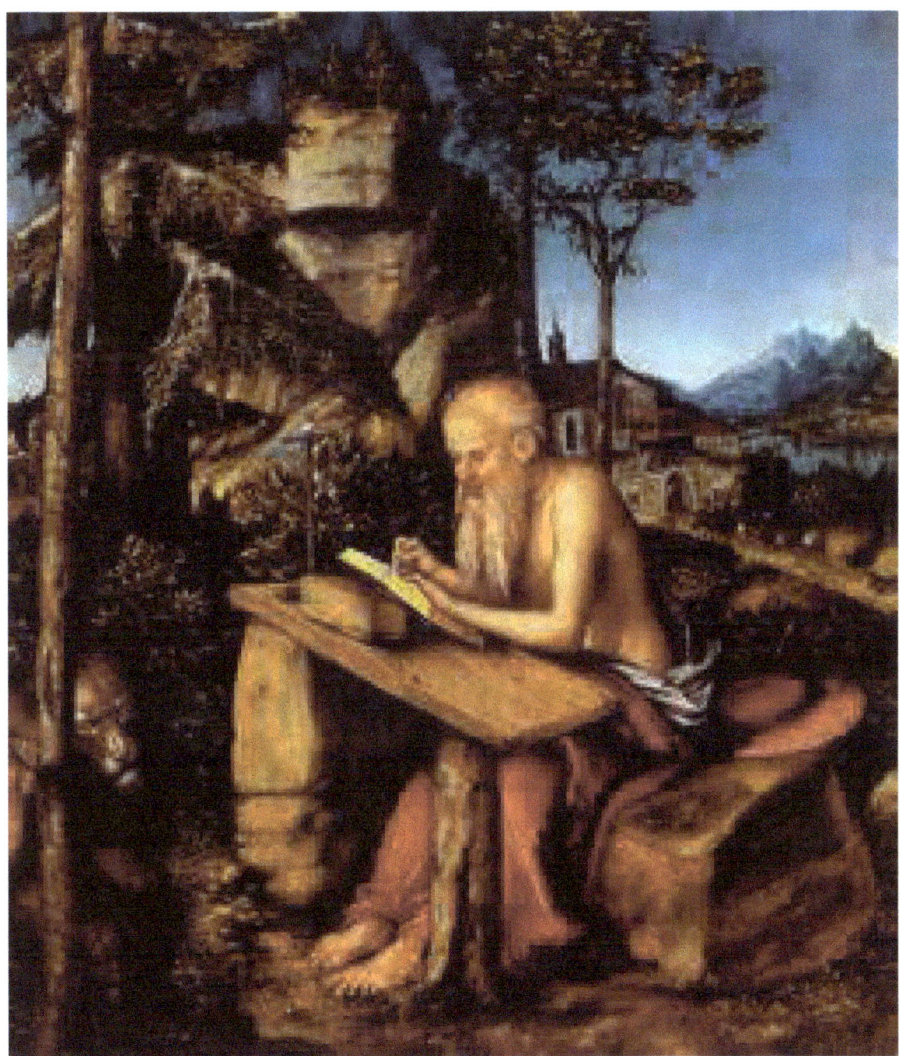
Saint Jerome Public Domain

Other Famous Quotes:

"Never look a gift horse in the mouth."
"Early impressions are hard to eradicate from the mind. When once wool has been dyed purple, who can restore it to its previous whiteness?"
"It is worse still to be ignorant of your ignorance."

Augustine of Hippo (St. Augustine)

Augustine of Hippo (St. Augustine) (354 AD – 430-AD) was a Christian philosopher and theologian. He was the bishop of Hippo Regius in present day Algeria. His approach generated the doctrine of original sin, and his writings included *City of God* and *Confessions*.

In his treatise on *City of God* he comments on the passing intestinal gas. He describes individuals that "have such command of their bowels, that they can break wind continuously at will, so as to produce the effect of singing".

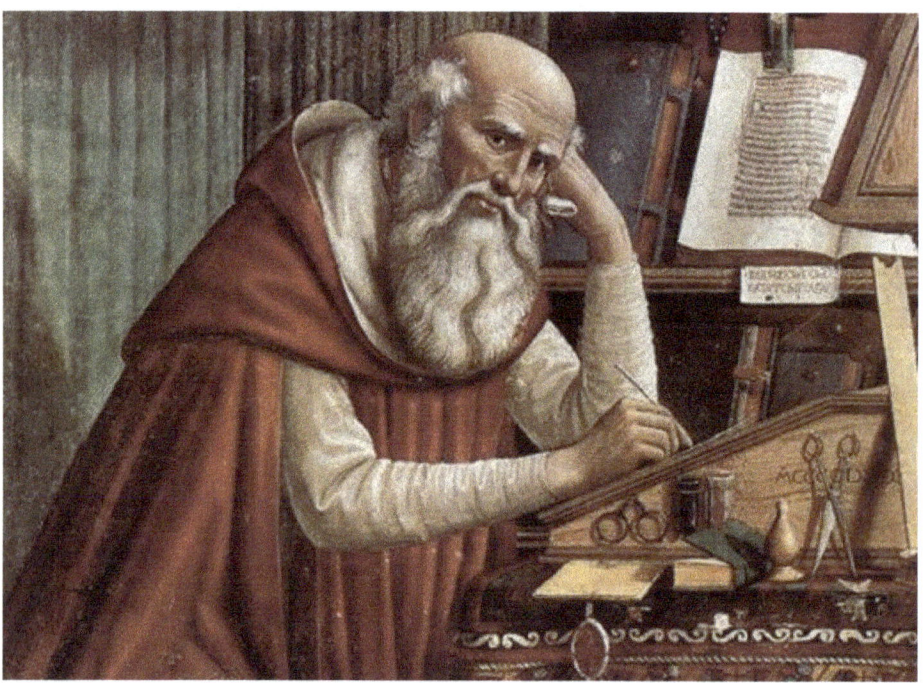

Augustine of Hippo (St. Augustine) Public Domain

Famous Quotations:

"Lord, Make me chaste, but not yet"
"Better to have loved and lost, than to have never loved at all."
"Complete abstinence is easier than perfect moderation."
"Patience is the companion of wisdom."
"Faith is to believe what we do not see; and the reward of this faith is to see what we believe."
"The World is a book, and those who do not travel read only a page."
"Seek not to understand that you may believe, but believe that you may understand."

Islam Hadith

In Islam the Hadith are writings of oral commentary that are ascribed to the teachings, sayings, and deeds of the Islamic prophet, Mohammed (c. 570 AD – 632 AD), may peace be upon him. They were collected often hundreds of years after the prophet lived. Many hadiths are not consistent with others, and there are continuing controversies within the branches of Islam as to which hadiths are truly authentic.

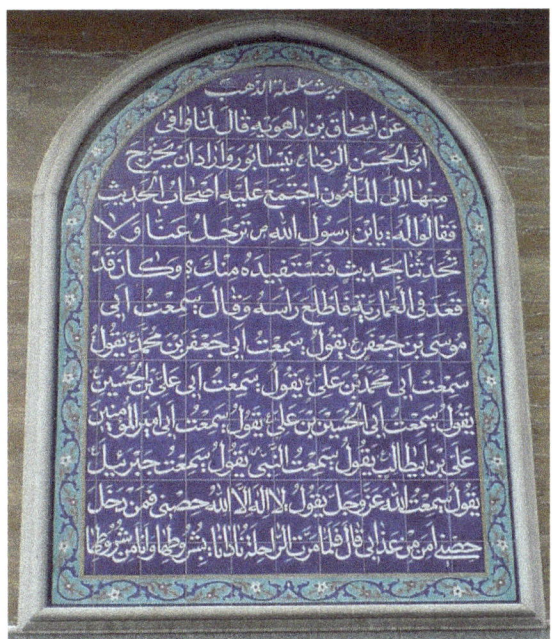

Hadith inscribed in Nishapur, Iran, Public Domain

Narrated Ali ibn Talq: The Apostle of Allah said: When any of you breaks wind during the prayer, he should turn away and perform ablution and repeat the prayer. *Abu Dawud* 1:205

Narrated 'Abbas bin Tamim: My uncle asked Allah's Apostle about a person who imagined to have passed wind during the prayer. Allah' Apostle replied: "He should not leave his prayers unless he hears sound or smells something. *"Sahih Bukhari* 1:4:139

Narrated Abu Huraira: The Prophet said, "Allah does not accept prayer of anyone of you if he does Hadath (passes wind) till he performs the ablution (anew)." *Sahih Bukhari* 9:86:86

Narrated 'Abdullah bin Zam'a: The Prophet forbade laughing at a person who passes wind. *Sahih Bukhari* 8:73:68

And Allah taught Adam all the names as follows: He taught him the name of everything, down to fart and little fart. *Tabari* 1:267

Istinja (Arabic: استنجاء), a component of Islamic hygiene practices, is the cleansing away of any residue and impurities (najasat) that remain after being passed from the urethra or anus. Istinja requires the use of water if available, and may be utilized with water alone or in combination with toilet paper. If water is not available stones, soil, or other natural material (other than bone or dung) may be utilized in the process known as 'istijmar'. The passage of intestinal gas alone does not require Istinja.

Sir Thomas Moore

Thomas Moore (1478 – 1535) was a philosopher, statesmen, theologian, and humanist who was subsequently canonized to sainthood by the Pope. King Henry VIII beheaded him when he refused to accept papal authority regarding his marriage to Catherine of Aragon.

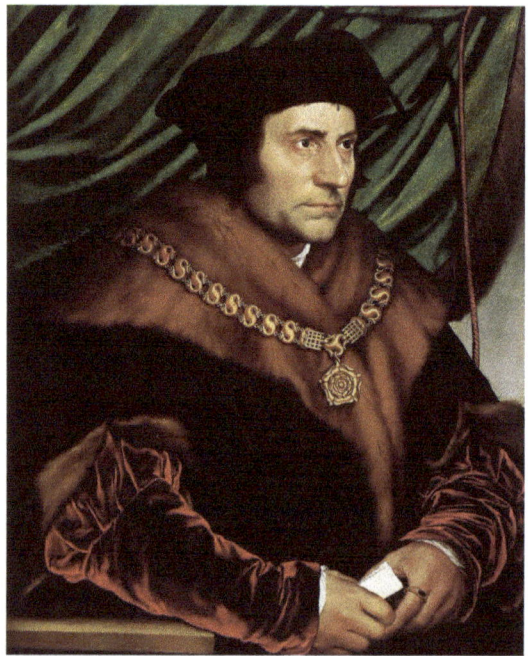

Portrait of Sir Thomas Moore 1527 by Hans Holbein the Younger in the Frick Collection, Google Art Project in the Public Domain

In 1518, Sir Thomas More, in an epigram entitled *In Efflatum Ventis*, wrote "'Wind, if you keep it too long in your stomach, kills you; on the other hand, it can save your life if it is properly let out. If wind can save or destroy you, then is it not as powerful as dreaded kings?'"

Famous Quotations:

To Them Who Trust in Fortune: None falleth far but he who climbeth high.

The Words of Fortune to the People: Better 'tis to be fortunate than wise!

Utopia: Man's folly hath enhanced the value of gold and silver because of their scarcity; whereas nature, like a kind parent, hath freely given us the best things, such as air, earth, and water, but hath hidden from us those which are vain and useless.

A Dialogue of Comfort Against Tribulation: I never saw fool yet that thought himself other than wise.

I die the King's good servant, but God's first.
— Last words on the scaffold, 1535 beheaded on order of King Henry VIII

Desiderius Erasmus

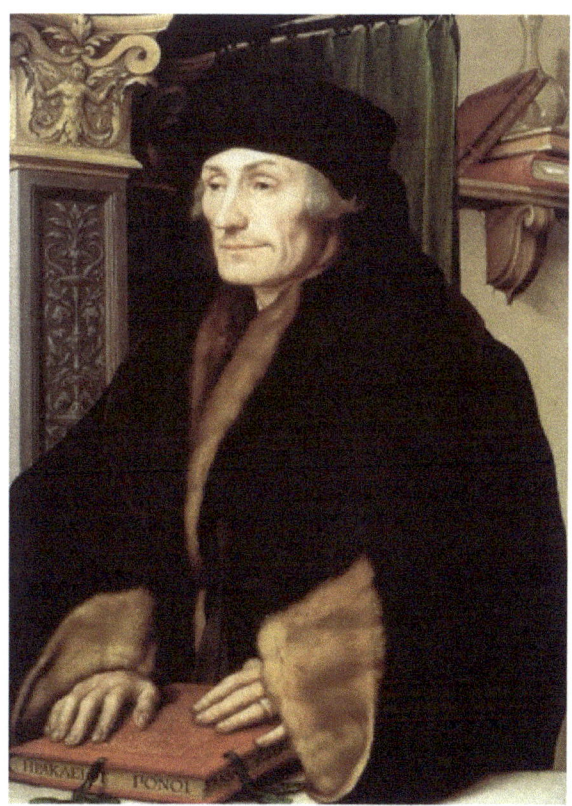

Portrait of Desiderius Erasmus of Rotterdam with Renaissance Pilaster in 1523 as depicted by Hans Holbein the Younger , National Gallery. Public Domain

Desiderius Erasmus Roterodamus (1466 – 1536) was a Dutch Renaissance humanist , classical scholar, social critic, teacher, and theologian who was an advocate for religious toleration.
His comments on farting include:

"Do not move back and forth on your chair. Doing so gives the impression of constantly breaking, or trying to break, wind."

"Retain the wind by compressing the belly.

Famous Quotations:

"The summit of happiness is reached when a person is ready to be what he is."
"In the land of the blind, the one-eyed man is king."
"The main hope of a nation lies in the proper education of its youth"
"If you keep thinking about what you want to do or what you hope will happen, you don't do it, and it won't happen."
"Before you sleep, read something that is exquisite, and worth remembering."
"He who allows oppression shares the crime."

Martin Luther

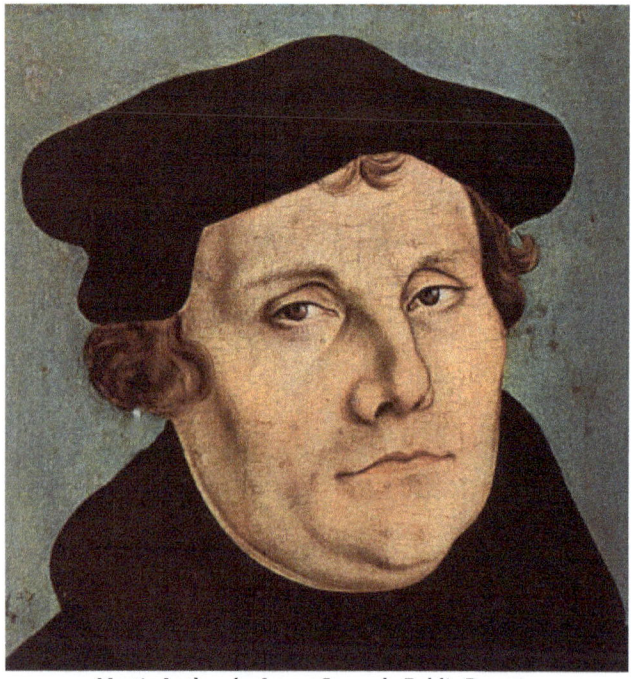

Martin Luther, by Lucas Cranach, Public Domain

Martin Luther (1483 – 1546) was a Catholic priest and German Monk who was a major figure in the Protestant Reformation. His confrontations with the Roman Catholic Church led to his excommunication.

He translated *The Bible* from Latin into German, and as a former priest decided to marry a former nun. He excoriated the Roman Catholic Church and anyone outside of his own closely held beliefs.

Although a major religious figure his published writings and letters, of which there are many, exhibit tendencies to embrace very earthy bodily functions. Farting appears to be one of his personal favorites and he described using his own prolific fart production to scare off the Devil on numerous occasions.

He also suffered from chronic constipation and spent a great deal of time on the toilet. He believed his intestinal problems were directly attributable to the Devil. The doctrine of justification by faith, the foundation on which the Protestant Reformation was based, came to him while in his usual repose, sitting on the toilet:

"This knowledge the Holy Spirit gave me on the privy in the tower" (quoted in Brown 202).

He also describes engaging in theological discussions with the devil and when his Lutheran doctrine did not suffice he blasted the devil 'mit einem Furz'."

"[S]hould some thought that isn't worth a fart nevertheless overwhelm me, I have the advantage (that our Lord God gives me) of taking hold of his Word once again." (Martin Luther, *Table Talk*, 461)

"Almost every night when I wake up the devil is there and wants to dispute with me. I have come to this conclusion: When the argument that the Christian is without the law and above the law doesn't help, I instantly chase him away with a fart." (Martin Luther, *Table Talk*, 469)

"Again, the Lord wants to have his sacrament given to strengthen the poor consciences through faith. 'No,' says pope fart-ass, 'one should sacrifice it for the dead and the living, sell it, and make a profitable business and market out of it so that we can expand our belly with it and devour all of the world's goods.'" (Martin Luther, *Against The Roman Papacy an Institution of the Devil*, 1545)

"I was frightened and thought I was dreaming, it was such a thunderclap, such a great horrid fart did the papal ass let go here! He certainly pressed with great might to let out such a thunderous fart—it is a wonder that it did not tear his hole and belly apart

If I were to ask here, 'But what did all the other apostles, especially St. Paul, pasture?' perhaps the big fart of the papal ass will say that maybe they pastured rats, mice, and lice, or, if it went well, sows, just so that the papal ass remains the shepherd, and all apostles swineherds." (Martin Luther, *Against The Roman Papacy an Institution of the Devil*, 1545)

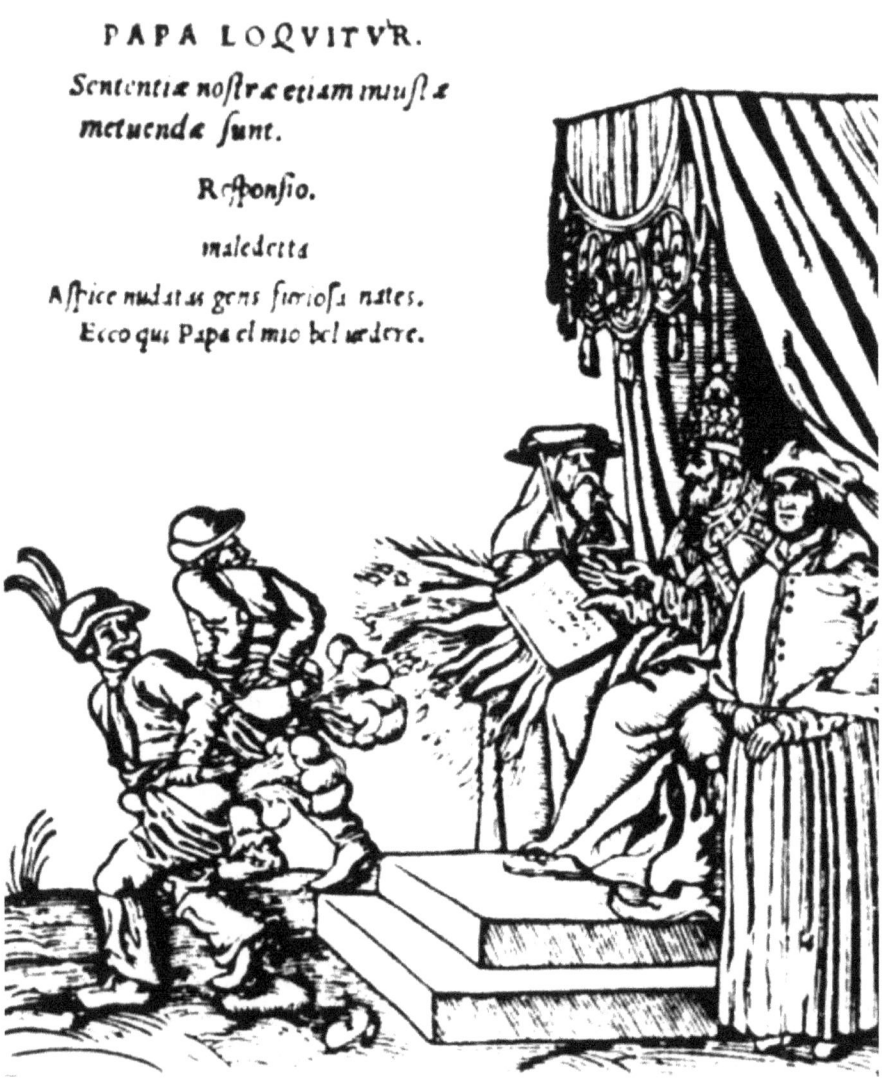

The Papal Belvedere by Lucas Cranach the Elder in the 1545 publication of Luther's Depiction of the Papacy. It features a papal bull complete with fire and brimstone, fresh from the hand of Pope Paul III meeting German peasants with farts, fresh from their "belvedere". Belvedere refers to a building in the Vatican, but also means "beautiful view". The Pope speaks: Our sentences are to be feared, even if unjust. Response: Be damned! Behold, o furious race, our bared buttocks. Here, Pope, is my 'belvedere' ,Public Domain.

"Again, the Lord wills that whoever confesses his sins and believes the absolution should be forgiven. 'No,' says ass-pope fart, 'faith does nothing; but your own repentance and atonement do, as well as the recounting of all your secret, forgotten, and unrecognized sins.' . . . The reason for this is that I have authority to bind and loose.

Perhaps even: 'Whoever does not worship my fart is guilty of a deadly sin and hell, for he does not acknowledge that I have the authority to bind and command everything. Whoever does not kiss my feet and, if I were to bind it so, lick my behind, is guilty of a deadly sin and deep hell, for Christ has given me the keys and authority to bind all and everything." (Martin Luther, *Against The Roman Papacy an Institution of the Devil*, 1545)

"This is the way—this is exactly the way one should lie and blaspheme if one wants to be a proper pope. Dear God, what an utterly shameless, blasphemous lying-mouth the pope is! He talks just as though no man on earth knew that the four principal councils and many others were held without the Roman church, and instead thinks like this, 'As I am a crude ass, and do not read the books, so there is no one in the world who reads them; rather, when I let my braying heehaw, heehaw resound, or even let out a donkey's fart, then everyone will have to consider it an article of faith; if not, St. Peter and St. Paul and God himself will be angry with them.'

For God is nowhere God anymore, except solely the assgod in Rome, where the big, crude asses (pope and cardinals) ride on better donkeys than they are." (Martin Luther, *Against The Roman Papacy an Institution of the Devil*, 1545)

"Why don't you fart nor burp? Wasn't the food to your liking?" The German version: "Warum furzet und rülpset ihr nicht? Hat es euch nicht geschmecket?" - sometimes it's "das Essen" instead of "es".

H.R.H. Queen Elizabeth I

Elizabeth I (1533 – 1603) was Queen of England from 1558 until her death. Her colorful reign, often referred to as the Elizabethan Era, had many luminaries interacting with her including William Shakespeare, Christopher Marlowe, Sir Francis Drake, Mary Queen of Scots and critical events such as the defeat of the Spanish Armada.

An apocryphal story is one of the Spanish Ambassador being presented to Queen Elizabeth I with what was anticipated to be a proposal to prevent hostilities. As the ambassador curtsied before the queen he released an inadvertent but audible, and perhaps pungent, release of gas. The coarse laughter and rebuke of his slippage so embarrassed and enraged the ambassador that he immediately withdrew and returned to Spain without making the proposal.

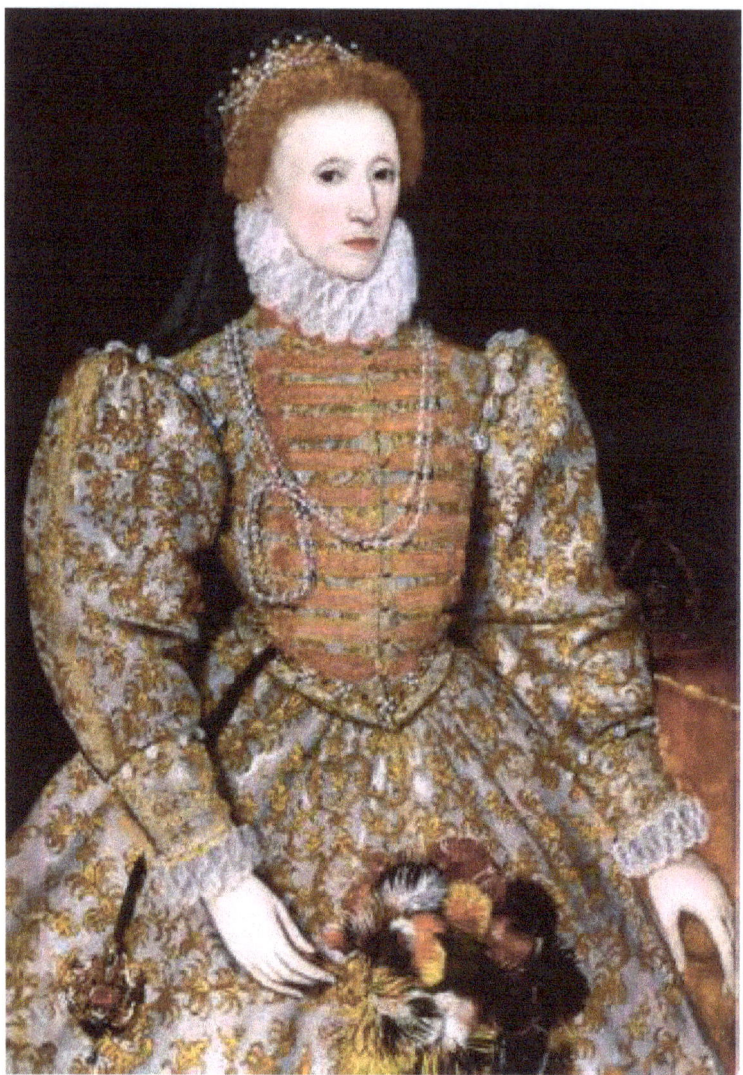

The Darnley Portrait of Elizabeth I of England. It was named after a previous owner. Probably painted from life, this portrait is the source of the face pattern called "The Mask of Youth" which would be used for authorized portraits of Elizabeth for decades to come. Recent research has shown the colors have faded. The oranges and browns would have been crimson red in Elizabeth's time. Artist Unknown, c. 1575 National Portrait Gallery London, Public Domain

The apocryphal story of the Spanish Ambassador is probably based on the following documented history recorded in the chronicles of the Royal Court. As per court protocol, Edward DeVere, the Earl of Oxford, was required to curtsy before Her Majesty the Queen. As he curtsied he accidently released a loud emanation. He had farted in front of Her Majesty and was so mortified he went into a self-imposed exile from the royal court for over ten years.

When he returned all those years later protocol required that he curtsy. Everyone anxiously waited, and he performed the requisite curtsy slowly, and showing great restraint, did not fart. He assumed that no one remembered the long ago fart, and that all was forgiven. Queen Elizabeth offered a sly pardon and said 'My Lord, I hath forgot the fart".

Famous Quotations:

"The past can not be cured."
"I observe and remain silent."
"Life is for living and working at. If you find anything or anybody a bore, the fault is in yourself."
"Do not tell secrets to those whose faith and silence you have not already tested."
"Men fight wars. Women win them."
"To be a king and wear a crown is a thing more glorious to them that see it than it is pleasant to them that bear it."
"There is no marvel in a woman learning to speak, but there would be in teaching her to hold her tongue"

Michel de Montaigne

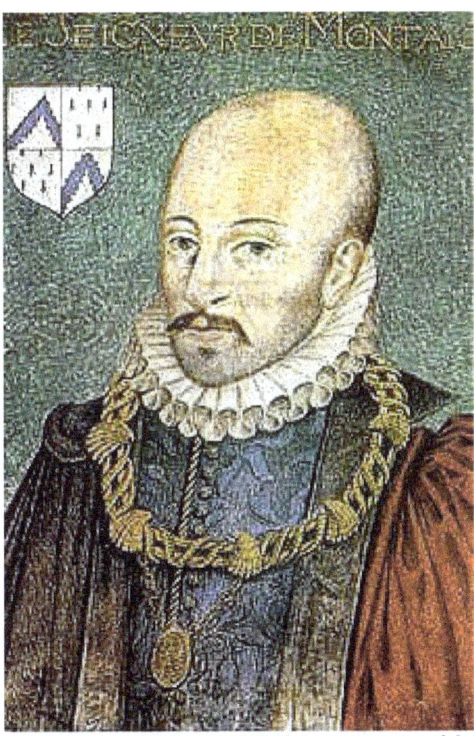

A portrait of Michel Eyquem de Montaigne (1533–1592) An engraving of this painting was published in the first edition of Montaigne's Essais, 1617. Public Domain

Artsy Fartsy: Cultural History of the Fart Volume One

Michel Eyquem de Montaigne (1533-1592) was a famed French Renaissance author, statesman, physician, essayist, and a long-term sufferer of chronic constipation.

"God alone knows how many times our bellies, by the refusal of one single fart, have brought us to the door of an agonizing death."

Famous Quotations:

"I am afraid that our eyes are bigger than our stomachs, and that we have more curiosity than understanding. We grasp at everything, but catch nothing except wind."
"Nothing is so firmly believed as that which we least know."
"The most certain sign of wisdom is cheerfulness. "
"On the highest throne in the world, we still sit only on our own bottom."
"If I speak of myself in different ways, that is because I look at myself in different ways."
"He who fears he shall suffer, already suffers what he fears."
"Nothing fixes a thing so intensely in the memory as the wish to forget it."
"Learned we may be with another man's learning: we can only be wise with wisdom of our own."
"Lend yourself to others, but give yourself to yourself."
"I do not care so much what I am to others as I care what I am to myself."
"I quote others only in order the better to express myself.
"When I am attacked by gloomy thoughts, nothing helps me so much as running to my books. They quickly absorb me and banish the clouds from my mind."
How many things served us yesterday for articles of faith, which today are fables for us?"
"There is nothing more notable in Socrates than that he found time, when he was an old man, to learn music and dancing, and thought it time well spent."
"To forbid us anything is to make us have a mind for it."
"I find I am much prouder of the victory I obtain over myself, when, in the very ardor of dispute, I make myself submit to my adversary's force of reason, than I am pleased with the victory I obtain over him through his weakness."
"I prefer the company of peasants because they have not been educated sufficiently to reason incorrectly."
"Obsession is the wellspring of genius and madness."
"Let us give Nature a chance; she knows her business better than we do."
"I speak the truth, not so much as I would, but as much as I dare; and I dare a little more as I grow older."
"If there is such a thing as a good marriage, it is because it resembles friendship rather than love."
"Off I go, rummaging about in books for sayings which please me."

Henry Ludlow

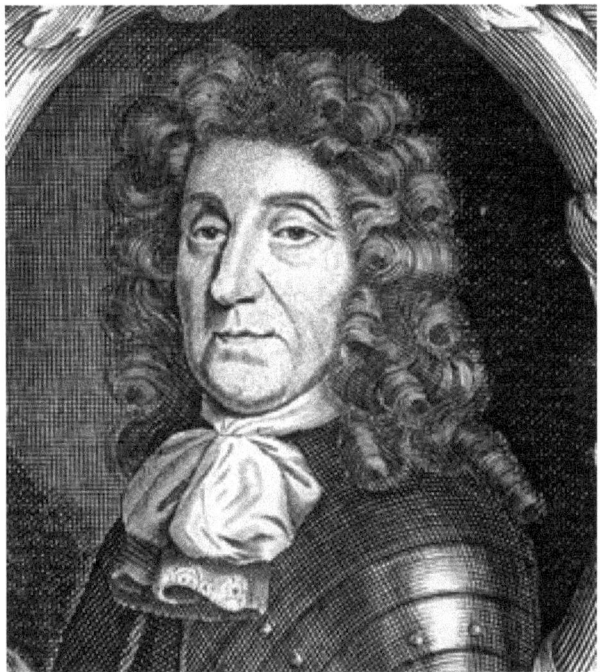

www.nndb.com/people Public Domain

Henry Ludlow (1577–1639), a Member of Parliament in England was participating in a vigorous debate about the naturalization of the Scots in 1607. When the roll call for votes was in process it was his turn to respond and everyone expected him to offer a resounding NAY!

Although it may have been an innocent accident since his father Sir Edward Ludlow was famous for having farted in a committee meeting, the resounding NAY emanated from his posterior. The House of Parliament fell into uproar and Ludlow's farting Nay-vote passed into posterity and folklore. Many poems were written about the fart, the best-known being the long winded *The Censure of the Parliament Fart* from the 1620's.

The Censure of the Parliament Fart

Never was bestowed such art
Upon the tuning of a Fart.
Downe came grave auntient Sir John Crooke1
And redd his message in his booke.
Fearie well, Quoth Sir William Morris, Soe:
But Henry Ludlowes Tayle cry'd Noe.
Up starts one fuller of devotion

Then Eloquence; and said a very ill motion
Not soe neither quoth Sir Henry Jenkin
The Motion was good; but for the stincking
Well quoth Sir Henry Poole it was a bold tricke
To Fart in the nose of the bodie pollitique
Indeed I must confesse quoth Sir Edward Grevill
The matter of it selfe was somewhat uncivill
Thanke God quoth Sir Edward Hungerford
That this Fart proved not a Turdd
Quoth Sir Jerome the lesse there was noe such abuse
Ever offer'd in Poland, or Spruce
Quoth Sir Jerome in folio, I swearer by the Masse
This Fart was enough to have brooke all my Glasse
Indeed quoth Sir John Trevor it gave a fowle knocke
As it lanched forth from his stincking Docke.
I (quoth another) it once soe chanced
That a great Man farted as hee danced.
Well then, quoth Sir William Lower
This fart is noe Ordinance fitt for the Tower.
Quoth Sir Richard Houghton noe Justice of Quorum
But would take it in snuffe to have a fart lett before him.

If it would beare an action quoth Sir Thomas Holcrofte
I would make of this fart a bolt, or a shafte.
Quoth Sir Walter Cope 'twas a fart rarely lett
I would 'tweere sweet enough for my Cabinett.
Such a Fart was never seene
Quoth the Learned Councell of the Queene.
Noe quoth Mr Pecke I have a President in store
That his Father farted the Session before
Nay then quoth Noy 'twas lawfully done
For this fart was entail'd from father to sonne
Quoth Mr Recorder a word for the cittie
To cutt of the aldermens right weere great pittie.
Well quoth Kitt Brookes wee give you a reason
Though he has right by discent he had not livery & seizing.

Ha ha quoth Mr Evans I smell a fee
I'ts a private motion heere's something for mee
Well saith Mr Moore letts this motion repeale
Whats good for the private is oft ill for comonweale
A good yeare on this fart, quoth gentle Sir Harry
He has caus'd such an Earthquake that my colepitts miscarry.

'Tis hard to recall a fart when its out
Quoth with a loude shooter

Oliver Cromwell

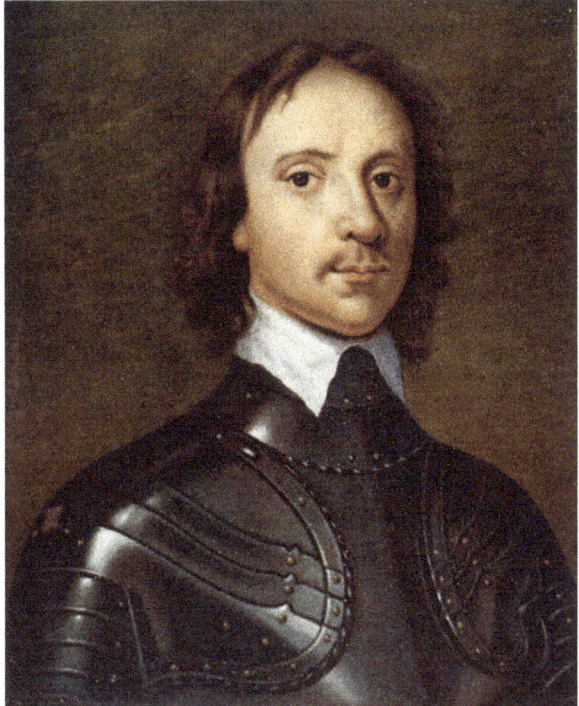
Oliver Cromwell, Public Domain

Oliver Cromwell (1599-1658) was a controversial English leader who has been variously labeled as a regicide, dictator, and hero of liberty. As a general with exceptional military prowess he was known as Old Ironsides. A member of Parliament he was instrumental in seeing that King Charles I was executed. An opposing lawyer made reference to the Magna Carta agreed to by King John of England in 1215. Cromwell's derogatory response was "I care not for the Magna Farta"
He dissolved parliament and rose to the leadership of the country as Lord Protector of England, Wales, Scotland, and Ireland. After his death from natural causes he was buried in Westminster Abbey. When Royalists returned to power his corpse was exhumed, hung in chains, and beheaded.

" I care not for the Magna Farta"

Lord John Wilmot, Earl of Rochester

Lord John Wilmot (1647 - 1680) Earl of Rochester was an English poet and satirist whose writings were frequently censored during the Victorian period.

Artsy Fartsy: Cultural History of the Fart Volume One

Lord John Wilmot, Earl of Rochester, Public Domain

He is the author of the following epistle:

Perhaps ill Verses, ought to be confined,
In mere good Breeding, like unsavory wind.
Were Reading forced, I should be apt to think
Men might no more write scurvily than stink.
But 'tis your choice, whether you'll read or no;
If likewise of your smelling it were so,
I'd Fart, just as I write, for my own ease,
Nor should you be concerned unless you please.

Famous Quotations:

"Before I got married I had six theories about raising children;
 now, I have six children and no theories."
"Here lies our sovereign lord the king,
Whose word no man relies on;
He never says a foolish thing,
Nor ever does a wise one."
"There's not a thing on earth that I can name,
So foolish, and so false, as common fame."
"Then Old Age, and Experience, hand in hand,
Lead him to death, and make him understand,
After a Search so painful, and so long,
That all his Life he has been in the wrong."

"Reason, an *Ignis fatuus* of the Mind,
Which leaves the light of Nature, Sense, behind."

Benjamin Franklin

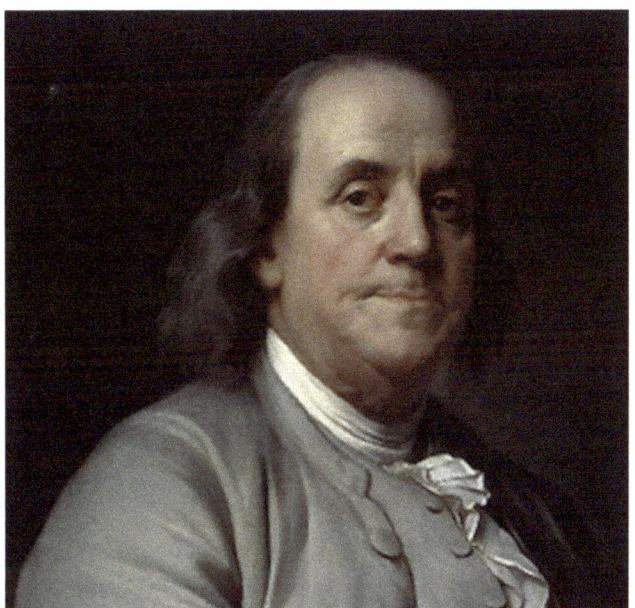

Portrait of Benjamin Franklin by Joseph Siffrein Duplessis c. 1785 National Portrait Gallery Washington D.C. Public Domain

Benjamin Franklin (1706-1790) was a polymath scientist, author, statesman, philosopher, publisher, diplomat, inventor, and humorist. In 1781 he was serving as the United States ambassador to France and with his scientific background kept in close communication with the European community of scientists. As is typical for a scientific congress an announcement from the Royal Academy of Brussels was made calling for the presentation of scientific papers on a host of subjects.

Franklin found some of the proposals so pretentious that his "bawdy, scurrilous nature" was stirred to compose a satirical response in the form of a proposal for research. As an illustrious statesman and scientist his proposal would demand serious attention.

"Let every fart count as a peal of thunder for liberty. Let every fart remind the nation of how much it has let pass out of its control. So fart, and if you must, fart often. But always fart without apology. Fart for freedom, fart for liberty… and fart proudly!"

His prolific writings on scatological subjects were published as a volume *Fart Proudly: Writings of Benjamin Franklin You Never Read in School*.

Artsy Fartsy: Cultural History of the Fart Volume One

"He that lives upon Hope, dies farting." is another of his famous quotes.

His proposal to the Royal Academy (reprinted in full below) called for scientific research to discover food additives that would provide a variety of attractive aromas to produce good smelling farts that would be socially welcomed.

To The Royal Academy of Brussels:

GENTLEMEN, I have perused your late mathematical Prize Question, proposed in lieu of one in Natural Philosophy, for the ensuing year, viz. "Une figure quelconque donnee, on demande d'y inscrire le plus grand nombre de fois possible une autre figure plus-petite quelconque, qui est aussi donnee".

I was glad to find by these following Words, "l'Acadeemie a jugee que cette deecouverte, en eetendant les bornes de nos connoissances, ne seroit pas sans UTILITE", that you esteem Utility an essential Point in your Enquiries, which has not always been the case with all Academies; and I conclude therefore that you have given this Question instead of a philosophical, or as the Learned express it, a physical one, because you could not at the time think of a physical one that promis'd greater Utility.

Permit me then humbly to propose one of that sort for your consideration, and through you, if you approve it, for the serious Enquiry of learned Physicians, Chemists, &c. of this enlightened Age. It is universally well known, That in digesting our common Food, there is created or produced in the Bowels of human Creatures, a great Quantity of Wind. That the permitting this Air to escape and mix with the Atmosphere is usually offensive to the Company, from the fetid Smell that accompanies it.

That all well-bred People therefore, to avoid giving such Offence, forcibly restrain the Efforts of Nature to discharge that Wind. That so retain'd contrary to Nature, it not only gives frequently great present Pain, but occasions future Diseases, such as habitual Cholics, Ruptures, Tympanies, &c. often destructive of the Constitution, & sometimes of Life itself. Were it not for the odiously offensive Smell accompanying such Escapes, polite People would probably be under no more Restraint in discharging such Wind in Company, than they are in spitting, or in blowing their Noses.

My Prize Question therefore should be, To discover some Drug wholesome & not disagreable, to be mix'd with our common Food, or Sauces, that shall render the natural Discharges of Wind from our Bodies, not only inoffensive, but agreeable as Perfumes. That this is not a chimerical Project, and altogether impossible, may appear from these Considerations. That we already have some Knowledge of Means capable of Varying that Smell.

He that dines on stale Flesh, especially with much Addition of Onions, shall be able to afford a Stink that no Company can tolerate; while he that has lived for some Time on Vegetables only, shall have that Breath so pure as to be insensible to the most delicate Noses; and if he can manage so as to avoid the Report, he may any where give Vent to his Griefs, unnoticed. But as there are many to whom an entire Vegetable Diet would be inconvenient, and as a little Quick-Lime thrown into a Jakes will correct the amazing Quantity of fetid Air arising from the vast Mass of putrid Matter contain'd in such Places, and render it rather pleasing to the Smell, who knows but that a little Powder of Lime (or some other thing equivalent) taken in our Food, or perhaps a Glass of Limewater drank at Dinner, may have the same Effect on the Air produc'd in and issuing from our Bowels?

This is worth the Experiment. Certain it is also that we have the Power of changing by slight Means the Smell of another Discharge, that of our Water. A few Stems of Asparagus eaten, shall give our Urine a disagreable Odour; and a Pill of Turpentine no bigger than a Pea, shall bestow on it the pleasing Smell of Violets. And why should it be thought more impossible in Nature, to find Means of making a Perfume of our Wind than of our Water? For the Encouragement of this Enquiry, (from the immortal Honour to be reasonably expected by the Inventor) let it be considered of how small Importance to Mankind, or to how small a Part of Mankind have been useful those Discoveries in Science that have heretofore made Philosophers famous.

Are there twenty Men in Europe at this Day, the happier, or even the easier, for any Knowledge they have pick'd out of Aristotle? What Comfort can the Vortices of Descartes give to a Man who has Whirlwinds in his Bowels! The Knowledge of Newton's mutual Attraction of the Particles of Matter, can it afford Ease to him who is rack'd by their mutual Repulsion, and the cruel Distensions it occasions? The Pleasure arising to a few Philosophers, from seeing, a few Times in their Life, the Threads of Light untwisted, and separated by the Newtonian Prism into seven Colours, can it be compared with the Ease and Comfort every Man living might feel seven times a Day, by discharging freely the Wind from his Bowels?

Especially if it be converted into a Perfume: For the Pleasures of one Sense being little inferior to those of another, instead of pleasing the Sight he might delight the Smell of those about him, & make Numbers happy, which to a benevolent Mind must afford infinite Satisfaction. The generous Soul, who now endeavours to find out whether the Friends he entertains like best Claret or Burgundy, Champagne or Madeira, would then enquire also whether they chose Musk or Lilly, Rose or Bergamot, and provide accordingly. And surely such a Liberty of Expressing one's Scent-iments, and pleasing one another, is of infinitely more Importance to human Happiness than that Liberty of the Press, or of abusing one another, which the English are so ready to fight & die for.

— In short, this Invention, if compleated, would be, as Bacon expresses it, bringing Philosophy home to Mens Business and Bosoms. And I cannot but conclude, that in Comparison therewith, for universal and continual UTILITY, the Science of the Philosophers above-mentioned, even with the Addition, Gentlemen, of your "Figure quelconque" and the Figures inscrib'd in it, are, all together, scarcely worth a FART-HING.

Artsy Fartsy: Cultural History of the Fart Volume One

Famous Quotations:

"Either write something worth reading or do something worth writing."
"Three may keep a secret, if two of them are dead."
"They who can give up essential liberty to obtain a little temporary safety deserve neither liberty nor safety."

"Tell me and I forget, teach me and I may remember, involve me and I learn."
"He that can have patience can have what he will."
"A penny saved is a penny earned"
"In wine there is wisdom, in beer there is Freedom, in water there is bacteria."
"You may delay, but time will not."
"Fear not death for the sooner we die, the longer we shall be immortal."
"Many people die at twenty five and aren't buried until they are seventy five."
"Never ruin an apology with an excuse."
"I didn't fail the test, I just found 100 ways to do it wrong."
"We are all born ignorant, but one must work hard to remain stupid."
"Justice will not be served until those who are unaffected are as outraged as those who are."
"How many observe Christ's birthday! How few, His precepts!"
"Hide not your talents, they for use were made,
What's a sundial in the shade?"
"By failing to prepare, you are preparing to fail."
"Well done is better than well said."
"Lost Time is never found again."
"Instead of cursing the darkness, light a candle."
"If all printers were determined not to print anything till they were sure it would offend nobody, there would be very little printed."
"Being ignorant is not so much a shame, as being unwilling to learn."
"The Constitution only guarantees the American people the right to pursue happiness. You have to catch it yourself."
"It is the first responsibility of every citizen to question authority."
"I am for doing good to the poor, but...I think the best way of doing good to the poor, is not making them easy in poverty, but leading or driving them out of it. I observed...that the more public provisions were made for the poor, the less they provided for themselves, and of course became poorer. And, on the contrary, the less was done for them, the more they did for themselves, and became richer."
"An investment in knowledge always pays the best interest."
"Be at war with your vices, at peace with your neighbors, and let every new year find you a better man."

Thomas Blount

Thomas Blount (1674 – 1681) an English lexicographer advised that 'Pease and beans are flatulent meat.' His principal work was *Glossographia; or, a dictionary interpreting the hard words of whatsoever language, now used in our refined*

English tongue (1656).

It defined approximately eleven thousand difficult or unusual words in the English language. It was the largest English dictionary in the world when it was published.

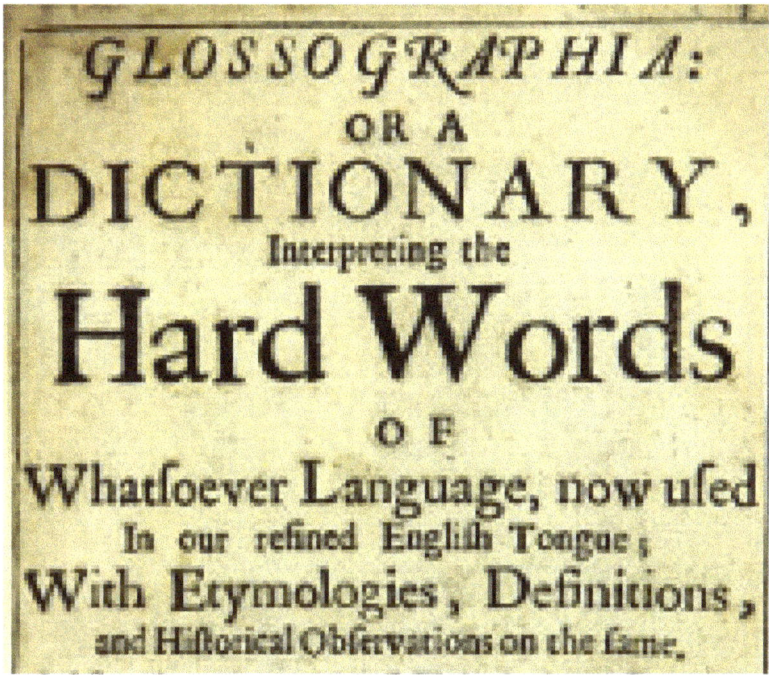

www.scricciolo.com/Nuovo_Neornithes/glossographia_gr. Public Domain

Famous Quotations:

Some will never learn anything because they understand everything too soon. As dreams are the fancies of those that sleep, so fancies are but the dreams of those awake.

Immanuel Kant

Immanuel Kant (1724 –1804) was a German Prussian philosopher. His work *Critique of Pure Reason* published in 1781 is often referred to as the beginning of modern philosophy.

Kant wrote a popular and scathing satire entitled the *Dreams of a Spirit-Seer* (1766). He denounces the philosopher Swedenborg as the "arch-spirit-seer of all spirit-seers", whose works are "fantasies"), "wild figments of the imagination", "eight tomes of nonsense", and the results of "hypochondrial winds".

Kant described these hypochondrial winds as farts when raging in the guts, and as heavenly visions when raging in the mind. Kant saw in the farting mystic a parody of himself.

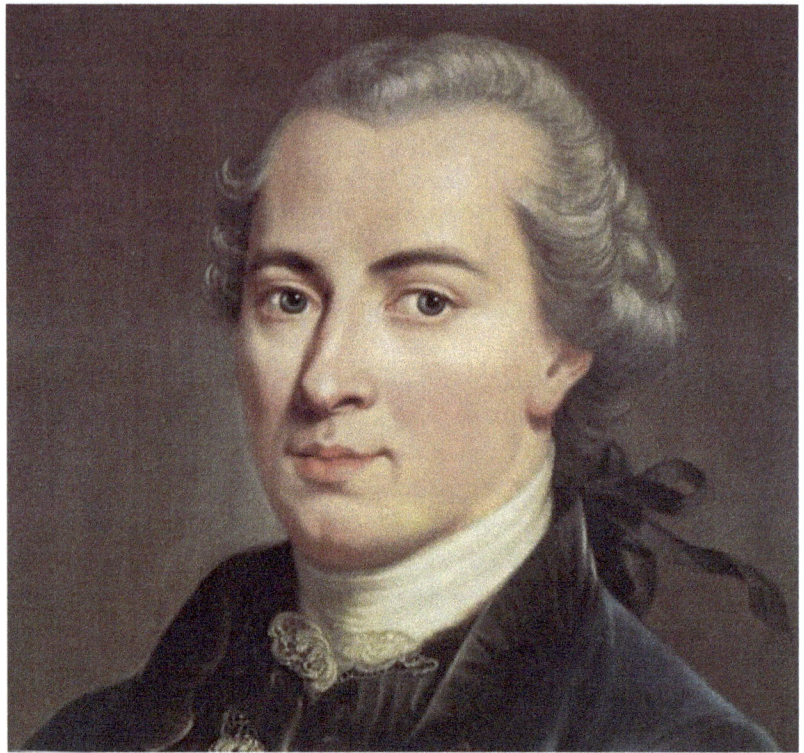

Immanuel Kant, Prussian philosopher. Public Domain

Famous Other Quotations:

"We are not rich by what we possess but by what we can do without."
"Science is organized knowledge. Wisdom is organized life. "
"All our knowledge begins with the senses, proceeds then to the understanding, and ends with reason. There is nothing higher than reason."
"He who is cruel to animals becomes hard also in his dealings with men. We can judge the heart of a man by his treatment of animals."
"Look closely. The beautiful may be small."
"For peace to reign on Earth, humans must evolve into new beings who have learned to see the whole first."
"The busier we are, the more acutely we feel that we live, the more conscious we are of life."
"The death of dogma is the birth of morality."
"High towers, and metaphysically-great men resembling them, round both of which there is commonly much wind, are not for me. My place is the fruitful bathos, the bottom-land, of experience; and the word transcendental, does not signify something passing beyond all experience, but something that indeed

precedes it a priori, but that is intended simply to make cognition of experience possible."

"Art is purposiveness without purpose."

"The whole interest of my reason, whether speculative or practical, is concentrated in the three following questions: What can I know? What should I do? What may I hope?

"The reading of all good books is like a conversation with the finest minds of past centuries."

"Enlightenment is the emancipation of man from a state of self-imposed tutelage... of incapacity to use his own intelligence without external guidance. Such a state of tutelage I call 'self-imposed' if it is due, not to lack of intelligence, but to lack of courage or determination to use one's own intelligence without the help of a leader. Sapere aude! Dare to use your own intelligence! This is the battle-cry of the Enlightenment."

"Laughter is an affect resulting from the sudden transformation of a heightened expectation into nothing."

"To be is to do."

"Experience without theory is blind, but theory without experience is mere intellectual play."

"it was the duty of philosophy to destroy the illusions which had their origin in misconceptions, whatever darling hopes and valued expectations may be ruined by its explanations."

Charles James Fox

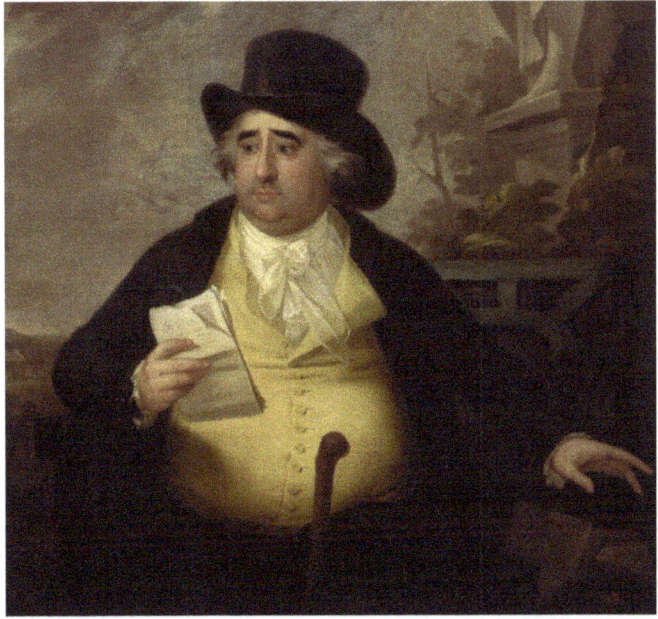

Charles James Fox, by Karl Anton Hickel National Portrait Gallery, Public Domain

Artsy Fartsy: Cultural History of the Fart Volume One

Charles James Fox (1749-1806) was a prominent member of the British Parliament and member of the Whig party. He was an outspoken critic of King George III and supported both the American and French Revolutions, as well as opposing slavery. His private life was considered colorful and notorious by the standards of the day.

Charles James Fox - *An Essay upon Wind* 1787

I have heard, from several of your brother peers, that your lordship farts, without reserve, when seated upon the woolsack, in a full assembly of nobles. This is honest and impartial in Your Lordship, and you merit the thanks of the nation at large... Now this is manly – I admire great Nature in all her operations, and detest the wretched affected being who would check or counteract her in any of her sublime and beautiful works.

Fame, my Lord, with her shrill loud trumpet, reports that Your Lordship's farts are as STRONG, and as SOUND, as your arguments – as VIGOROUS as your intellects – as FORCIBLE as your language – as BRILLIANT as your wit – and as SONOROUS and MUSICAL as Your Lordship's voice... May Your Lordship continue to fart like an ancient Grecian for many years. For those who he anticipated resentful approbation he went so far as to include a humorously self-deprecating introduction.

"I think I hear the CURIOUS reader exclaim, 'Heavens! That the brain of a man should be set to work on such cursed nonsense - such damned low stuff as farting; he ought to be ashamed of straining his dull facilities to such a nasty, absorb subject. But to PRINT his THOUGHTS upon farting, and to dedicate his dirty lucubrations to the Lord Chancellor, is the height of all human impudence and folly.'"

"I take it there are five or six different species of farts, and which are perfectly distinct from each other, both in weight and smell. First, the sonorous and full-toned, or rousing fart; Second, the double fart; Third, the soft fizzing fart; fourth, the wet fart; and Fifth, the sullen wind-bound fart."

To add to the discussion it was sure to generate the pamphlet opens with the following epigraph, courtesy of John Wilmont, 2d Earl of Rochester:
Perhaps such writing ought to be confined
In mere good breeding, like unsavory wind.
Were reading forced, I should be apt to think,
Men might no more write scurvily than stink:
But 'tis your choice whether you'll read or no;
If likewise of your smelling, it were so,
I'd fart, just as I write, for in my own ease,
Nor should you be concerned unless you please.

Abraham Lincoln

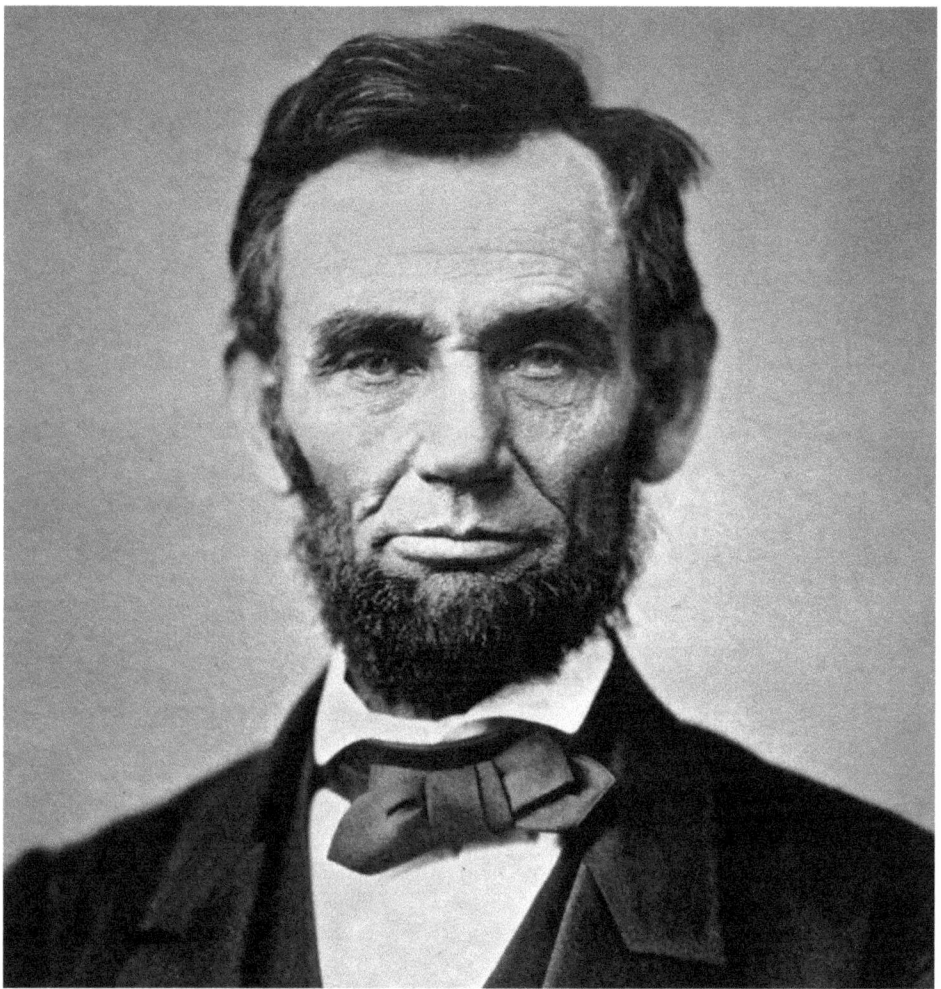

Abraham Lincoln, sixteenth United States President 1863 daguerreotype Author Alexander Gardner, Public Domain

Abraham Lincoln (1809 – 1865) was the 16th President of the United States, statesman and philosopher. He was known for his fondness for off color stories and earthy sense of humor. When asked in 1859 why he did not publish a book of his collected stories he made a face as if encountering a horrible stench and said "Such a book would stink like a thousand privies. " As recounted in the two-volume *Abraham Lincoln: A Life* by Michael Burlingame the following stories are written verbatim with their original grammar and spelling of the time.

Lincoln told of a "man of audacity, quick witted, self-possessed, & equal to all occasions" who was given the honor and task to carve a turkey for a large party.

"The men and women surrounded the table & the audacious man being chosen to carver whetted his great carving knife with the steel and got down to business & commenced carving the turkey, but he expended too much force & let a fart—a loud fart so that all the people heard it distinctly.

As a matter of course it shocked all terribly. A deep silence reigned. However the audacious man was cool & entirely self possessed; he was curiously & keenly watched by those who knew him well, they suspecting that he would recover in the end and acquit himself with glory.

The man with a kind of sublime audacity, pulled off his coat, rolled up his sleeves—put his coat deliberately on a chair—spat on his hands—took his position at the head of the table—picked up the carving knife & whetted it again, never cracking a smile nor moving a muscle of his face. It now became a wonder in the minds of all the men & women how the fellow was to get out of his dilemma; he squared himself and said loudly & distinctly—'Now by God I'll see if I can't cut up this turkey without farting.' "

Abner Ellis recalled this Lincoln story: "It appears that Shortly after we had pease with England Mr. [Ethan] Allen had occasion to visit England, and while their the English took Great pleasure in teasing him, and trying to Make fun of the Americans and General Washington in particular and one day they got a picture of General Washington, and hung it up in the Back House.

Mr. Allen Could see it and they finally asked Mr A if he saw that picture of his friend in the Back House. Mr Allen said no. but said he thought that it was a very appropriate [place] for an Englishman to keep it[.] Why they asked. For said Mr Allen there is Nothing that will make an Englishman Shit So quick as the Sight of Genl Washington."

"When I was a little boy," he once said, "I lived in the state of Kentucky, where drunke[n]ness was very co[m]mon on election days. At an election…in a village near where I lived, on a day when the weather was inclement and the roads exceedingly muddy, A Toper named Bill got brutally drunk and staggered down a narrow alley where he layed himself down in the mud, and remained there until the dusk of the evening, at which time he recovered from his stupor. Finding himself very muddy, [he] immediately started for a pump (a public watering-place on the street) to wash himself[.]

On his way to the pump another drunken man was leaning over a horse post[;] this, Bill mistook for the pump and at once took hold of the arm of the man for the handle, the use of which set the occupant of the post throwing up.

Bill believing all was right put both hands under and gave himself a thorough washing. He then made his way to the grocery for something to drink. On entering the door one of his comrades exclaimed in a tone of surprise, Why Bill what in the world is the matter[?] Bill said in reply by G-d you ought to have seen me before I washed."

Lincoln told the story about a fellow "who had a great veneration for Revolutionary relics. He heard tha[t] an old lady…had a dress which she had worn in the Revolutionary war. He made a special visit to this lady and asked her if she could produce the dress as a satisfaction to his love of aged things. She obliged him by opening a drawer and bringing out the article in question.

The enthusiastic person took up the dress and delivered an apostrophe to it, 'Were you the dress,' said he, 'that this lady once young and blooming wore in the time of Washington? No doubt when you came home from the dress maker she kissed you as I do now!' At this the relic hunter took the old dress and kissed it heartily. The practical old lady rather resented such foolishness over an old piece of wearing apparel and she said: 'Stranger if you want to kiss something old you had better kiss my ass. It is sixteen years older than that dress."

Famous Quotations:

"Most folks are about as happy as they make their minds up to be."
"It has been my experience that folks who have no vices have very few virtues."
"No man is good enough to govern another man without that other's consent."
"Better to remain silent and be thought a fool, than to speak and remove all doubt."
"Always bear in mind that your own resolution to succeed, is more important than any other one thing."
"My great concern is not whether you have failed, but whether you are content with your failure."
"If I had eight hours to chop down a tree, I'd spend six hours sharpening my ax"
"I destroy my enemies when I make them my friends."
"You cannot strengthen the weak by weakening the strong."
"Those who deny freedom to others deserve it not for themselves."
"I have always found that mercy bears richer fruits that strict justice."
"Books serve to show a man that those original thoughts of his aren't very new after all"
"If you call a tail a leg, how many legs has a dog? Five? No, calling a tail a leg don't make it a leg."
"A house divided against itself cannot stand."
"Be sure you put your feet in the right place, then stand firm."
"With the fearful strain that is on me night and day, if I did not laugh I should die"
"I walk slowly, but I never walk backward"
"Democracy is the government of the people, by the people, for the people"
"I can make a General in five minutes but a good horse is hard to replace."
"What is conservatism? Is it not adherence to the old and tried, but against the new and untried"

"A statesman is he who thinks in the future generations, and a politician is he who thinks in the upcoming elections."

"In the end it is not the years in your life that count. It is the life in your years"
"Whatever you are, be a good one."
"The philosophy of the school room in one generation will be the philosophy of government in the next."
"You can have anything you want - if you want it badly enough. You can be anything you want to be, do anything you set out to accomplish if you hold to that desire with singleness of purpose."
"I don't like that man. I must get to know him better."
"If I am killed, I can die but once; but to live in constant dread of it, is to die over and over again"
"Towering genius disdains a beaten path. It seeks regions hitherto unexplored."
"The best way to get a bad law repealed is to enforce it strictly."
"You may deceive all the people part of the time, and part of the people all the time, but not all the people all the time."
"I'm sorry I wrote such a long letter. I did not have the time to write a short one."
"No man has a good enough memory to make a successful liar."
"Truth is generally the best vindication against slander"
"If I were two faced, would I be wearing this one?"
"I do not think much of a man who is not wiser today than he was yesterday."
"He reminds me of the man who murdered both his parents, and then when sentence was about to be pronounced pleaded for mercy on the grounds that he was an orphan"
"He can compress the most words into the smallest idea of any man I know"
"Freedom is the last, best hope of earth."
"Every one desires to live long, but no one would be old.
"Human action can be modified to some extent, but human nature cannot be changed."
"Sorrow comes to all...Perfect relief is not possible, except with time. You cannot now realize that you will ever feel better and yet you are sure to be happy again."
"When I do good, I feel good. When I do bad, I feel bad. That's my religion."
"Whenever I hear anyone arguing for slavery, I feel a strong impulse to see it tried on him personally."
"You cannot escape the responsibility of tomorrow by evading it today."
"The best thing about the future is that it comes only one day at a time."
"Things may come to those who wait...but only the things left by those who hustle."
"Government of the people, by the people, for the people, shall not perish from the Earth."
"We should be too big to take offense and too noble to give it."
"You cannot build character and courage by taking away a man's initiative and independence."
"I fear explanations explanatory of things explained"

Sir Richard Burton

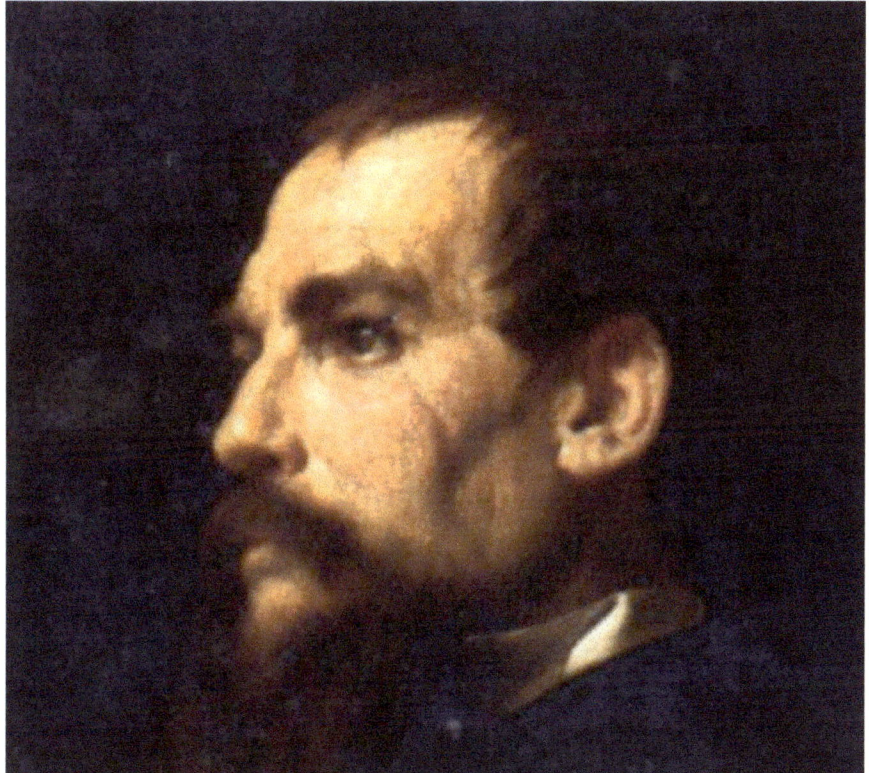
Richard Burton, 1875 by Frederic Leighton. Public Domain

Captain Sir Richard Francis Burton (1821 – 1890) was an English geographer, translator, orientalist, explorer, translator, cartographer, writer, diplomat, soldier, ethnologist, spy, linguist, poet, and fencer. He was known for his extraordinary facility and knowledge of languages and cultures. He insinuated himself into the heart of Arabic culture and was one of the few westerners who travelled to Mecca incognito. He was the translator of *The Arabian Nights*, and related the tale of the unforgettable fart of Abu al-Hassan, The Merchant of Oman tale.

"He let fly two great farts, one of which blew up the dust from the earth's face and the other steamed up the gates of Heaven." Abu – al-Hassan upon his wedding night "let fly a fart, great and terrible". He was so ashamed he ran from house and went into exile for ten years. When re returned, hoping that his fart was long forgotten he overheard a mother telling her child she "was born on the very night that Abu al-Hassan farted!" Mortified that his fart had become a landmark day in the history of his people he returned to exile never to return gain.

He also described that the even inadvertent passage of a fart, or the embarrassment of someone else who farted, could easily lead to the literal loss of one's head in the fury of the protection of honor at all costs. One of his scholarly footnotes observes that the wild onion of Tibet, 'the only procurable green-stuff, produces an odor so rank and fetid that men run away from their own crepitation.'

Releasing intestinal gas either as a burp or belch (itkerreh) or as a fart (zirt) was considered by the Arabs as an act of purification as it drove unclean and all evil spirits from the body. A very loud fart (Zirt) was acceptable behavior in the presence of others and the generator would be fondly referred to as Abu ez-Zirteh (Father of the Fart).

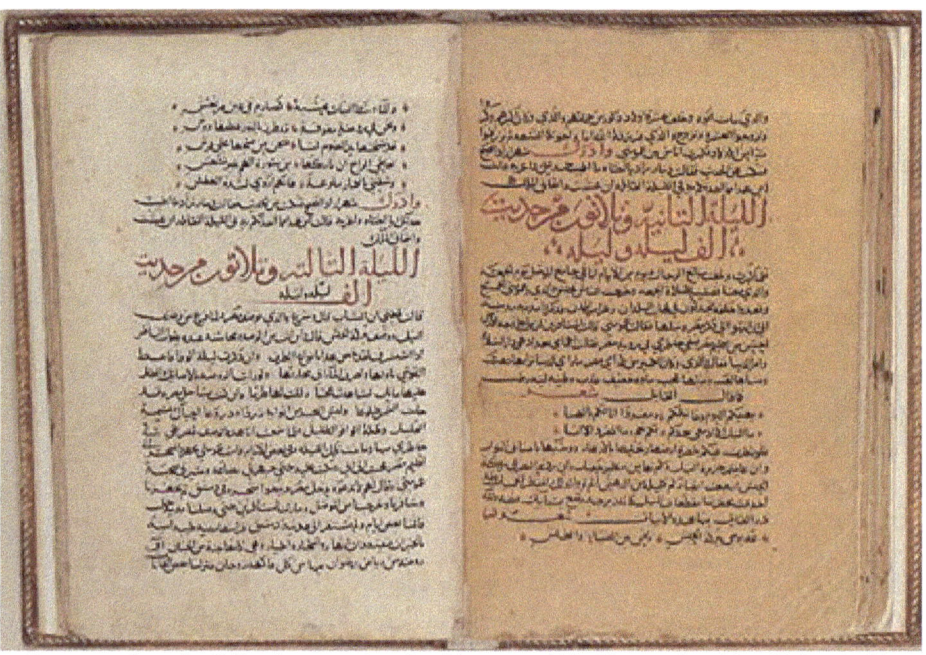

Two pages from the Galland manuscript, the oldest text of *The Thousand and One Nights*. Arabic manuscript, back to the 14th century from Syria. Public Domain

A silent but deadly variety of fart, also known in English as a fizzle (faswah) was as offensive as the stench and was considered an inflammatory insult. The fizzler was referred to as Fezwaun but no word was given to describe the recipient of the aromatic airs.

Reportedly the release of intestinal gas, particularly in the presence of royalty, was given an immediate capital punishment and quite a number of Arabs died because either they passed the culprit or were unfairly blamed for someone else's release.

It may well have been that having the ability to maintain a poker face well before the creation of the card game could save one's life if they could bluff that the person next to them was the scoundrel. The sense of smell was much stronger than a sense of humor as even laughing at the passing of gas could lead to an immediate killing to preserve the honor of the farter. In that culture at that time killer farts were all too real and the penalty for trespass unforgiving.

Here are his original footnote comments: Alluding to the curious phenomenon pithily expressed in the Latin proverb, "Suus cuique crepitus bene olet," I know of no exception to the rule, except amongst travellers in Tibet, where the wild onion, the only procurable green-stuff, produces an odour so rank and fetid that men run away from their own crepitations.

The subject is not savoury, yet it has been copiously illustrated: I once dined at a London house whose nameless owner, a noted bibliophile, especially of "facetiae," had placed upon the drawing-room table a dozen books treating of the "Crepitus ventris." When the guests came up and drew near the table, and opened the volumes, their faces were a study.

Another version of these folk tales was compiled and published as *The Book of the Thousand Nights and One Night* in 1923 by Edward Powys Mathers. The story that follows was entitled *The Father of Farts*.

That morning the girl prepared a dish consisting of beans, peas, white haricots, cabbage, lentils, onions, and cloves of garlic, various heavy grains and powdered spices. The qadi's enormous belly was quite empty when he returned for the midday meal, so he took helping after helping of this mixture, until all was finished...

The qadi congratulated himself, as he had so often done before, on the excellent choice of a wife; but an hour afterwards his belly began visibly to swell. A noise as of a far-off tempest made itself heard inside him. Low grumblings and far thunders shook the walls of his being and brought in their train sharp colics, spasms, and a final agony. He grew yellow in the face and began to roll groaning about the floor, holding his belly in his two hands.

"Allah, Allah!" he cried. "I have a terrible storm within! Who will deliver me?" Soon his paunch became as tight as a gourd, and his cries brought his wife running. She made him swallow a powder of anise and fennel, which was soon to have its effect, and, at the same time, to console and encourage him, began rubbing and patting the afflicted part, as if he had been a little sick child...

Then his pains increased, and he fell howling to the floor in a crisis of agony. Suddenly came relief. A long and thunderous fart broke from him, shaking the foundations of the house and throwing its utterer violently forward, so that he swooned. Then followed a multitude of other escapes, gradually diminishing in sound but rolling and re-echoing through the troubled air. Last came a single deafening explosion, and all was still.

Famous Quotations:

"Do what thy manhood bids thee do, from none but self expect applause. He noblest lives and noblest dies who makes and keeps his self-made laws."
"The more I study religions the more I am convinced that man never worshipped anything other than himself."

John Gregory Bourke

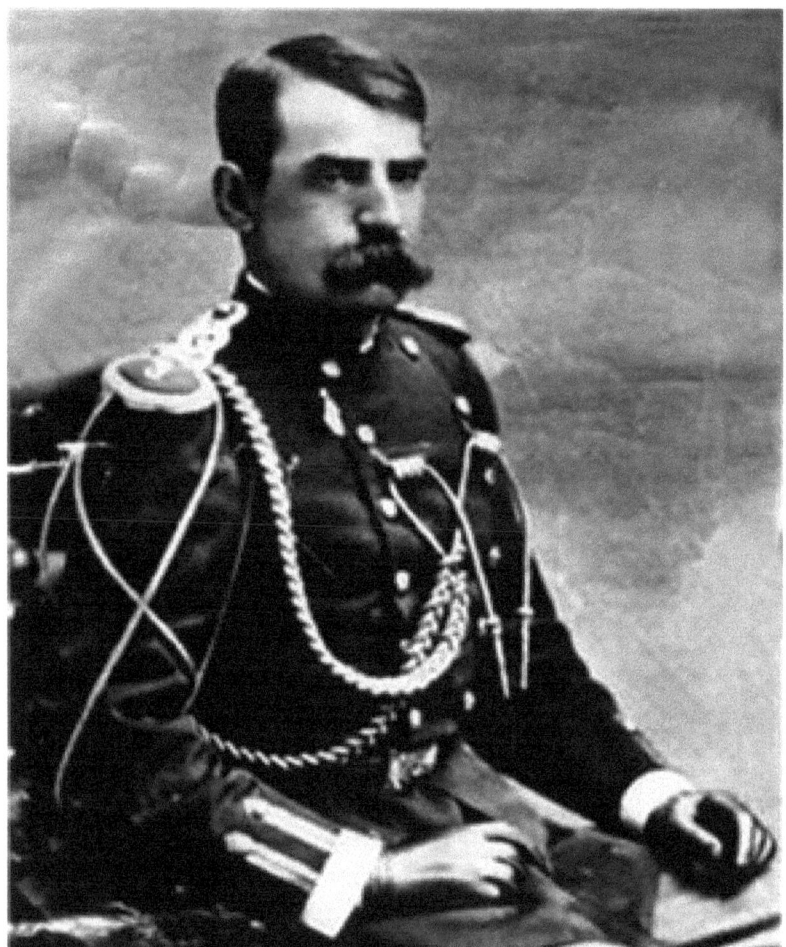

United States military captain, John Gregory Bourke (1843-1896) American Anthropologist, Public Domain

John Gregory Bourke (1843 – 1896) was a captain in the United States Army as well as a prolific diarist and postbellum author. He authored several books about the American Old West, including ethnologies of its indigenous peoples.

He spent a decade of his scientific career actively performing field research on scatological, urological, and sexual folklore and rites for his book *Scatological Rites of All Nations.* Even today over one hundred years later it makes for a fascinating read both from a cultural anthropology perspective as well as a humanitarian one. With the advent of electronic books is that a scanned copy of this volume, and other post copyright classics are available online on sites that are complimentary as well as some sites that are fee based.

His classic five hundred and sixteen page magnum opus work has been digitized from the Yale University Medical Library and is available online. The history and extent of religious, cultural, ethnic, and dietary use of both human and animal excrement is remarkable in its worldwide distribution.

" Their Beetle-gods out of their privies yea, their Privies and Farts had their unsavorie canonization and went for Egyptian deities. ... So, Hierome derideth their dreadfull deitie, the Onion, and a stinking Fart, Crepitus ventris inflati que Pelusiaco religio est, which they worshipped at Pelusium."

" The ancient Pelusiens, a people of lower Egypt, did (amongst other whimsical, chimerical objects of veneration and worship) venerate a Fart, which they worshipped under the symbol of a swelled paunch." — (*A View of the Levant* by Charles Perry, M. D., sm. fob, London, 1743, p. 419.

SCATALOGIC RITES

OF ALL NATIONS.

A Dissertation upon the Employment of Excrementitious Remedial Agents in Religion, Therapeutics, Divination, Witchcraft, Love-Philters, etc., in all Parts of the Globe.

BASED UPON ORIGINAL NOTES AND PERSONAL OBSERVATION, AND UPON COMPILATION FROM OVER ONE THOUSAND AUTHORITIES.

Scatalogic Rites of All Nations A Dissertation upon the Employment of Excrementitious Remedial Agents in Religion, Therapeutics, Divination, Witchcraft, Love-Philters, etc., in all Parts of the Globe by Captain John G. Bourke, U. S. A., Public Domain

It may be well to bear in mind that the heathen idea of the power of a god was entirely different from our own. The deities of the heathen were restricted in their powers and functions ; they were assigned to the care of certain countries, districts, valleys, rivers, fountains, etc. Not only that, they were capable of aiding only certain trades, professions, etc. They were not able to cure all diseases, only particular kinds, each god being a specialist; consequently, each was supposed to take charge of a section of the human body.

This was the case with the Greeks, Romans, Egyptians, and others. In mediaeval times the same rule obtained, only in place of gods, we find saints assigned to these functions. Saint Erasmus was in charge of "the belly, with the entrayles." Saint Phiacre would be prayed to for relief "of the phyoremeroids (hemorrhoids), of those especially which grow in the fundament."

Keeping this in view, we can better understand the peculiar ceremonies connected with the worship of Bel-Phegor; he was, no doubt, the deity to whom the devotee resorted for the alleviation of ailments connected with the rectum and belly.

On the same principle that the worshipper was wont to hang up in the temples of Esculapius wax and earthen representations of the sore arms, legs, and other members which gave him pain, the worshipper of Bel-Phegor would offer him the sacrifice of the flatulence and excrement, testimonies of the good health for which gratitude was due to the older deity.

Sigmund Freud

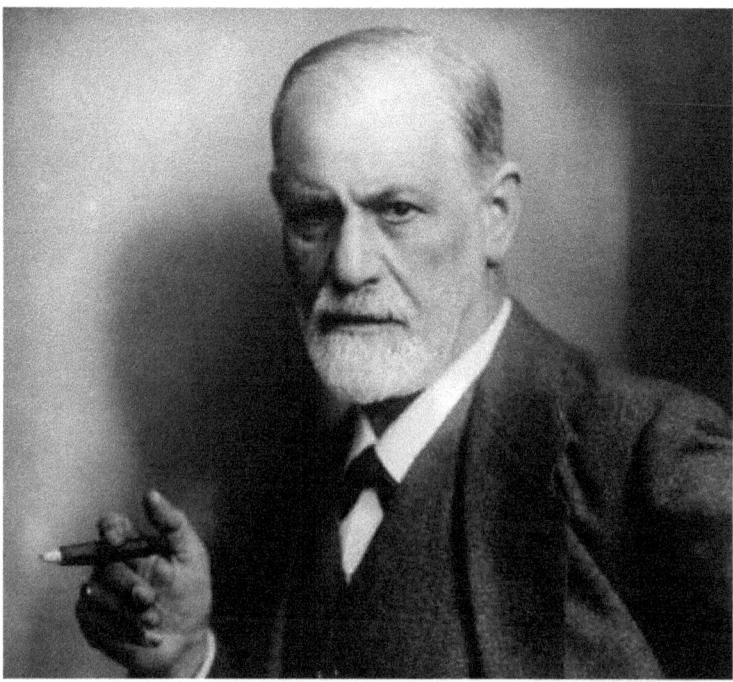

Sigmund Freud, founder of psychoanalysis,. Photographer Max Halberstadt) Public Domain

Sigismund Schlomo Freud (1856 – 1939) was an Austrian neurologist considered the founding father of psychoanalysis in psychiatry. His work is replete with references to anal, phallic, and oral fixation issues.

Freud considered a variety of physical symptoms as comprising the syndrome of neurasthenia, a condition no longer recognized as a physical ailment. At the beginning of the twentieth century it was commonly diagnosed in young American women and nicknamed Americanitis.

Its symptoms included fatigue, dyspepsia with flatulence, and indications of intra-cranial pressure and spinal irritation. He believed to neurasthenia to be due to "non-completed coitus", and therapy was aimed at achieving orgasmic release of nervous tension. The treatment of providing orgasmic release was very popular in medical practice in the early twentieth century.

The doctors and nurses providing this service were complaining that the service was resulting in their hands becoming overly fatigued. The development and popularization of the electrical massager and vibrator has been directly attributed to the demands of the medical professional.

For many years access to these devices was limited to licensed medical practices. When they became available to the general public, their popularity increased further. Home remedy for neurasthenia could now be accomplished in the privacy of the home without the expense or embarrassment requiring an appointment with and assistance of a doctor or nurse.

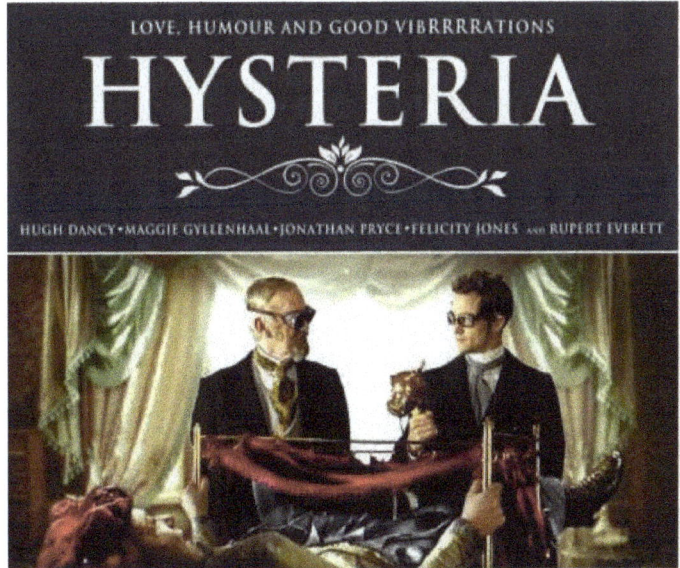

www.film.com/movie/-hysteria

Artsy Fartsy: Cultural History of the Fart Volume One

The romantic comedy movie *Hysteria* released in 2012 provides some additional background on this remarkable story. For a detailed review of the vibrator in medical history *The Technology of Orgasm* by Rachel Maines, Johns Hopkins University Press makes for a fascinating and provocative read. This is as good a place as any in this volume to mention that a vaginal fart, commonly called a queef, is also a normal physiological event and has also found its way into the literature movies, and even television.

Famous Quotations:

"We are never so defenseless against suffering as when we love."
"Unexpressed emotions will never die. They are buried alive and will come forth later in uglier ways."
"In the depths of my heart I can't help being convinced that my dear fellow-men, with a few exceptions, are worthless."
"It is impossible to escape the impression that people commonly use false standards of measurement — that they seek power, success and wealth for themselves and admire them in others, and that they underestimate what is of true value in life."
"Religion is a system of wishful illusions together with a disavowal of reality, such as we find nowhere else but in a state of blissful hallucinatory confusion. Religion's eleventh commandment is "Thou shalt not question."
"Religion is an illusion and it derives its strength from the fact that it falls in with our instinctual desires."
"Words have a magical power. They can bring either the greatest happiness or deepest despair; they can transfer knowledge from teacher to student; words enable the orator to sway his audience and dictate its decisions. Words are capable of arousing the strongest emotions and prompting all men's actions."
"The madman is a dreamer awake"
"When making a decision of minor importance, I have always found it advantageous to consider all the pros and cons. In vital matters, however, such as the choice of a mate or a profession, the decision should come from the unconscious, from somewhere within ourselves. In the important decisions of personal life, we should be governed, I think, by the deep inner needs of our nature."
"The more the fruits of knowledge become accessible to men, the more widespread is the decline of religious belief."
"Where id is, there shall ego be"
"What progress we are making. In the Middle Ages they would have burned me. Now they are content with burning my books. "
"The creative writer does the same as the child at play; he creates a world of fantasy which he takes very seriously."
"Men are more moral than they think and far more immoral than they can imagine."
"Properly speaking, the unconscious is the real psychic; its inner nature is just as

unknown to us as the reality of the external world, and it is just as imperfectly reported to us through the data of consciousness as is the external world through the indications of our sensory organs."
"Dreams are the royal road to the unconscious."
"The unconscious of one human being can react upon that of another without passing through the conscious."
 "In matters of sexuality we are at present, every one of us, ill or well, nothing but hypocrites."
"The first human who hurled an insult instead of a stone was the founder of civilization."
"When one does not have what one wants, one must want what one has."
"Sometimes a cigar is just a cigar."
"Dreams are often most profound when they seem the most crazy."

T.E. Lawrence of Arabia

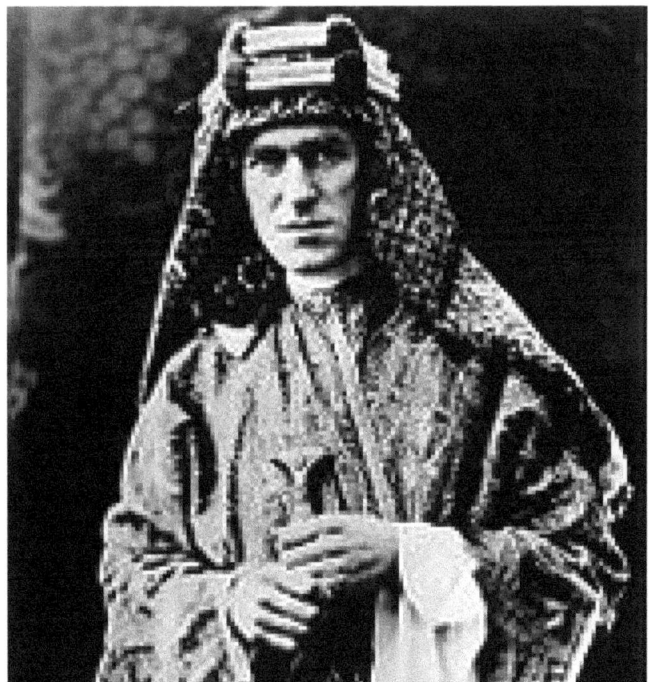

Lieutenant Colonel Thomas Edward Lawrence 1919 Photo by Lowell Thomas published in With Lawrence in Arabia in the Public Domain

T. E. Lawrence (1888 – 1935) of Lawrence of Arabia fame describes his introduction to an Arabian mealtime custom in his book *The Seven Pillars of Wisdom*. When he was about to join a festive meal with his Bedouin hosts another British officer pulled him aside to share an important gesture of gratitude.

He was strongly advised that if he did not loudly burp and belch during the course of the meal that they would be offended that he did not appreciate their hospitality. One might assume, quite wrongly, that an eruption from the other orifice would also be a sign of appreciation.

Famous Quotations:

"All men dream: but not equally. Those who dream by night in the dusty recesses of their minds wake up in the day to find it was vanity, but the dreamers of the day are dangerous men, for they may act their dreams with open eyes, to make it possible."
"Mankind has had ten-thousand years of experience at fighting and if we must fight, we have no excuse for not fighting well."
"The printing press is the greatest weapon in the armory of the modern commander."

Sir Winston Churchill

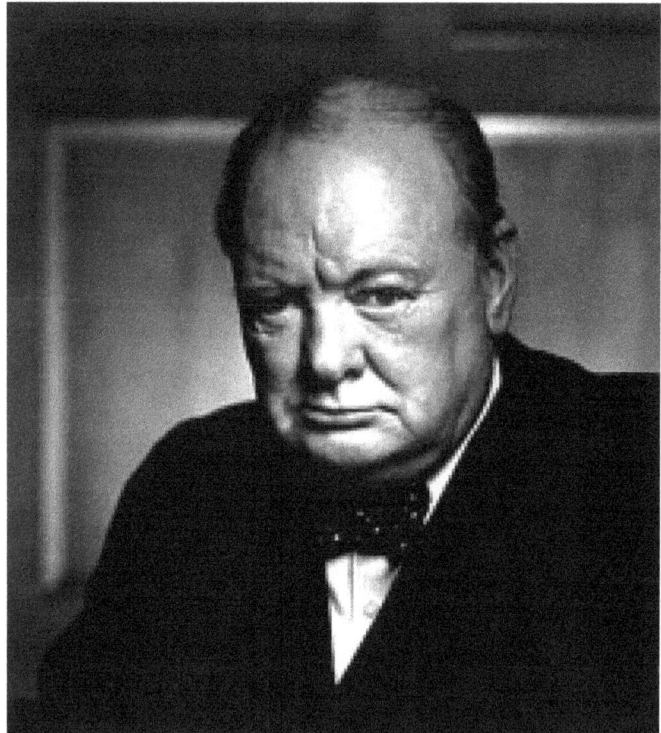

Sir Winston Churchill, Public Domain

Sir Winston Leonard Spencer Churchill (1874-1965) was a British statesmen and Prime Minister during the Second World War. He was also an accomplished artist, historian and author. He won the Nobel Prize in Literature.

Artsy Fartsy: Cultural History of the Fart Volume One

The apocryphal exchange took place at a dinner party where Sin Winston Churchill farted audibly. An offended gentleman reproached him saying "How dare you pass wind in front of my wife!" Sir Winston's response was "I am sorry, I did not know it was her turn."

Famous Quotations:

"Short words are best, and old words when short are best of all."
"Churchill was in the lavatory in the House of Commons and his secretary knocked on the door and said: Excuse me Prime Minister, but the Lord Privy Seal wishes to speak to you. After a pause Churchill replied: Tell His Lordship: I'm sealed on The Privy and can only deal with one shit at a time"
"A pessimist sees the difficulty in every opportunity; an optimist sees the opportunity in every difficulty."
"My tastes are simple: I am easily satisfied with the best."
"If you are going through hell, keep going."
"Tact is the ability to tell someone to go to hell in such a way that they look forward to the trip."
"Success is stumbling from failure to failure with no loss of enthusiasm."
"Personally, I'm always ready to learn, although I do not always like being taught."
"Never give in. Never give in. Never, never, never, never—in nothing, great or small, large or petty—never give in, except to convictions of honour and good sense. Never yield to force. Never yield to the apparently overwhelming might of the enemy."
"The greatest lesson in life is to know that even fools are right sometimes."
"We make a living by what we get. We make a life by what we give."
"He has all the virtues I dislike and none of the vices I admire."
"Continuous effort - not strength or intelligence - is the key to unlocking our potential."
"All the great things are simple, and many can be expressed in a single word: freedom, justice, honor, duty, mercy, hope"
"Diplomacy is the art of telling people to go to hell in such a way that they ask for directions."
"We make a living by what we get, but we make a life by what we give.
"The inherent vice of capitalism is the unequal sharing of blessings; the inherent virtue of socialism is the equal sharing of miseries."
"We contend that for a nation to tax itself into prosperity is like a man standing in a bucket and trying to lift himself up by the handle."
"The whole history of the world is summed up in the fact that, when nations are strong, they are not always just, and when they wish to be just, they are no longer strong."
"Courage is what it takes to stand up and speak;
Courage is also what it takes to sit down and listen."
"What is the use of living, if it be not to strive for noble causes and to make this muddled world a better place for those who will live in it after we are gone?"
"Of course I am an egoist, where do you get if you aren't?"

"My education was interrupted only by my schooling."
"Money is like manure, its only good if you spread it around."
"People stumble over the truth from time to time,
but most pick themselves up and hurry off as if nothing happened."
"Never, give in! Never give in! Never, never, never… In nothing great or small, large or petty, never give in except to convictions or honor and good sense!"
"You can always count on the Americans to do the right thing, after they have exhausted all the other possibilities."
"I am ready to meet my Maker. Whether my Maker is prepared for the ordeal of meeting me is another matter."
"It has been said that democracy is the worst form of government except all the others that have been tried."
"As one's fortunes are reduced, one spirit must expand to fill the void."
"Socialism is a philosophy of failure, the creed of ignorance, and the gospel of envy, its inherent virtue is the equal sharing of misery."
"It matters very little whether your judgments of people are true or untrue, and very much whether they are kind or unkind,"
"Success is not final, failure is not fatal: it is the courage to continue that counts"
"The inherent vice of capitalism is the unequal sharing of blessings; the inherent virtue of socialism is the equal sharing of miseries."
"I like pigs. Dogs look up to us. Cats look down on us. Pigs treat us as equals."
"A modest man with much to be modest about"
"History will be kind to me, for I intend to write it."
"We are all worms, but I do believe that I am a glow-worm."
"One must never forget when misfortunes come that it is quite possible they are saving one from something much worse; or that when you make some great mistake, it may very easily serve you better than the best-advised decision. Life is a whole, and luck is a whole, and no part of them can be separated from the rest."
"I cannot forecast to you the action of Russia. It is a riddle, wrapped in a mystery, inside an enigma; but perhaps there is a key. That key is Russian national interest."
"I am certainly not one of those who need to be prodded. In fact, if anything, I am the prod."
"The empires of the future are the empires of the mind."
"It is one thing to see the forward path and another to be able to take it. But it is better to have an ambitious plan than none at all."
"Let us learn our lessons. Never, never, never believe any war will be smooth and easy, or that anyone who embarks on that strange voyage can measure the tides and hurricanes he will encounter. The Statesman who yields to war fever must realise that once the signal is given, he is no longer the master of policy but the slave of unforeseeable and uncontrollable events."
"By swallowing evil word unsaid no one has ever yet harmed his stomach."
"Nothing in life is so exhilarating as to be shot at without result"
"Those who fail to learn from history are doomed to repeat it."
"Lady Nancy Astor: Winston, if you were my husband, I'd poison your tea. Churchill: Lady Astor, if I were your husband, I'd drink it."

"The fact that in Mohammedan law every woman must belong to some man as his absolute property – either as a child, a wife, or a concubine – must delay the final extinction of slavery until the faith of Islam has ceased to be a great power among men. Individual Moslems may show splendid qualities. Thousands become the brave and loyal soldiers of the Queen; all know how to die; but the influence of the religion paralyses the social development of those who follow it. No stronger retrograde force exists in the world. Far from being moribund, Mohammedanism is a militant and proselytizing faith. It has already spread throughout Central Africa, raising fearless warriors at every step; and were it not that Christianity is sheltered in the strong arms of science – the science against which it had vainly struggled – the civilization of modern Europe might fall, as fell the civilization of ancient Rome."

"What shall I do with all my books? was the question; and the answer, Read them, sobered the questioner. But if you cannot read them, at any rate handle them and, as it were, fondle them. Peer into them. Let them fall open where they will. Read on from the first sentence that arrests the eye. Then turn to another. Make a voyage of discovery, taking soundings of uncharted seas. Set them back on your shelves with your own hands. Arrange them to your own plan, so that if you do not know what is in them, you at least know where they are. If they cannot be your friends, let them at any rate be your acquaintances."

"Churchill: "Madam, would you sleep with me for five million pounds?"
Socialite: "My goodness, Mr. Churchill... Well, I suppose, of course... "
Churchill: "Would you sleep with me for five pounds?"
Socialite: "Mr. Churchill, what kind of woman do you think I am?!" Churchill: "Madam, we've already established that. Now we are haggling about the price"

Adolf Hitler

Adolf Hitler (1889 – 1945) was the Austrian born leader of the National Socialist (Nazi) Party, Chancellor of Germany and dictator (Führer) of Nazi Germany during the Second World War. According to Pulitzer Prize winning historian and biographer John Toland, "suffered from meteorism, uncontrollable farting".

To deal with this very embarrassing and uncomfortable (especially for those in his close proximity) condition Hitler was first prescribed Dr. Koster's anti-gas pills in 1936. By 1941 he was ingesting between "one hundred and twenty to one hundred and fifty anti-gas pills a week". In 1943 his physician Theodor Morell wrote in his diary that Hitler had "constipation and colossal flatulence on a scale I have seldom encountered before".

Three years later Dr. Erwin Giesling became Hitler's new physician and on examining the pills "was horrified to learn they contained strychnine and atropine". The side effects of these two toxic products include delirium, hallucinations, and paranoia. Whether his anti-flatulent therapy contributed to his sociopathic, megalomania, and mental instability is unknown.

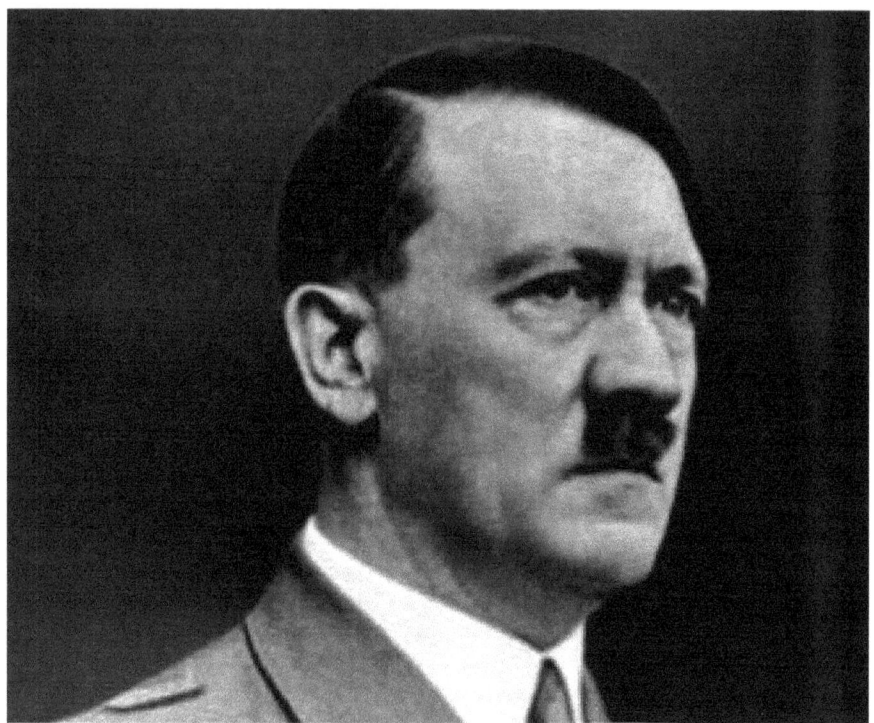

Adolf Hitler 1937 German Federal Archives llgemeiner Deutscher Nachrichtendienst - Zentralbild Bundesarchive Public Domain

Famous Quotations:

"If you win, you need not have to explain...If you lose, you should not be there to explain!"
"If you tell a big enough lie and tell it frequently enough, it will be believed."
"What luck for rulers that men do not think."
"Think a thousand times before taking a decision. But after taking a decision never turn back, even if you get a thousand difficulties!!"
"Anyone can deal with victory. Only the mighty can bear defeat."
"Those who want to live, let them fight, and those who do not want to fight in this world of eternal struggle do not deserve to live."
"It is not truth that matters, but victory."
"Great liars are also great magicians."
"By the skillful and sustained use of propaganda, one can make a people see even heaven as hell or an extremely wretched life as paradise."
"I do not see why man should not be as cruel as nature"
The man who has no sense of history, is like a man who has no ears or eyes"

"He alone, who owns the youth, gains the future."
"Demoralize the enemy from within by surprise, terror, sabotage, assassination. This is the war of the future."
"I use emotion for the many and reserve reason for the few."
"Who says I am not under the special protection of God?"
"The art of reading consists in remembering the essentials and forgetting non essentials."
"Kill, Destroy, Sack, Tell lies as much you want, after victory nobody asks why?"
To conquer a nation, first disarm its citizens."
"The victor will never be asked if he told the truth. "
The very first essential for success is a perpetually constant and regular employment of violence."
"The great masses of the people will more easily fall victims to a big lie than to a small one."
"Humanitarianism is the expression of stupidity and cowardice."
"Woman's world is her husband, her family, her children and her home. We do not find it right when she presses into the world of men."
"Anyone who sees and paints a sky green and fields blue ought to be sterilized."
"My spirit will rise from the grave and the world will see I was right."
"To the Christian doctrine of the infinite significance of the individual human soul and of personal responsibility, I oppose with icy clarity the saving doctrine of the nothingness and insignificance of the individual human being, and of his continued existence in the visible immortality of the nation"."
"Winning without problem is just victory ,
but winning with lots of trouble create History .."
"There is a better chance of seeing a camel pass through the eye of a needle than of seeing a really great man 'discovered' through an election."
"No politician should ever let himself be photographed in a bathing suit."
"The state must declare the child to be the most precious treasure of the people. As long as the government is perceived as working for the benefit of the children, the people will happily endure almost any curtailment of liberty and almost any deprivation."
"Struggle is the father of all things. It is not by the principles of humanity that man lives or is able to preserve himself above the animal world, but solely by means of the most brutal struggle."
"I believe today that my conduct is in accordance with the will of the Almighty."
"The best way to take control over a people and control them utterly is to take a little of their freedom at a time, to erode rights by a thousand tiny and almost imperceptible reductions. In this way, the people will not see those rights and freedoms being removed until past the point at which these changes cannot be reversed."
"Life doesn't forgive weakness."
"The application of force alone, without support based on a spiritual concept, can never bring about the destruction of an idea or arrest the propagation of it, unless one is ready and able to ruthlessly to exterminate the last upholders of that idea even to a man, and also wipe out any tradition which it may tend to leave behind."

"Sparta must be regarded as the first völkisch state. The exposure of the sick, weak, deformed children, in short, their destruction, was more decent and in truth a thousand times more human than the wretched insanity of our day which preserves the most pathological subject."
"Conscience is a Jewish invention."
"This year will go down in history. For the first time, a civilized nation has full gun registration. Our streets will be safer, our police more efficient, and the world will follow our lead into the future!"
"Truly, this earth is a trophy cup for the industrious man. And this rightly so, in the service of natural selection. He who does not possess the force to secure his Lebensraum in this world, and, if necessary, to enlarge it, does not deserve to possess the necessities of life. He must step aside and allow stronger peoples to pass him by."
"I know that fewer people are won over by the written word than by the spoken word and that every great movement on this earth owes its growth to great speakers and not to great writers."

"Our strength consists in our speed and in our brutality. Genghis Khan led millions of women and children to slaughter—with premeditation and a happy heart. History sees in him solely the founder of a state. It's a matter of indifference to me what a weak western European civilization will say about me. I have issued the command—and I'll have anybody who utters but one word of criticism executed by a firing squad—that our war aim does not consist in reaching certain lines, but in the physical destruction of the enemy. Accordingly, I have placed my death-head formation in readiness—for the present only in the East—with orders to them to send to death mercilessly and without compassion, men, women, and children of Polish derivation and language. Only thus shall we gain the living space (Lebensraum) which we need. Who, after all, speaks to-day of the annihilation of the Armenians?"

"My feeling as a Christian points me to my Lord and Savior as a fighter. It points me to the man who once in loneliness, surrounded only by a few followers, and who, God's truth! was greatest not as a sufferer but as a fighter. In boundless love as a Christian and as a man I read through the passage which tells us how the Lord at last rose in His might. Today, after two thousand years, with deepest emotion I recognize more profoundly than ever before the fact that it was for this that He had to shed his blood upon the Cross."

The receptivity of the masses is very limited, their intelligence is small, but their power of forgetting is enormous. In consequence of these facts, all effective propaganda must be limited to a very few points and must harp on these in slogans until the last member of the public understands what you want him to understand by your slogan."

"I don't see much future for the Americans ... it's a decayed country. And they have their racial problem, and the problem of social inequalities ... my feelings against

Americanism are feelings of hatred and deep repugnance ... everything about the behaviour of American society reveals that it's half Judaised, and the other half negrified. How can one expect a State like that to hold together?"

Josef Stalin

Widely regarded to be one of the most villainous leaders in history, Josef Stalin (1878-1953) was born as Ioseb Besarionis dze Dzhugashvili. He ruled the Soviet Union with an iron fist from the mid-1920s until his death in 1953. The number of people who died as a result of his policies that many consider genocide or pathological paranoia is conservatively estimated at over twenty five million.

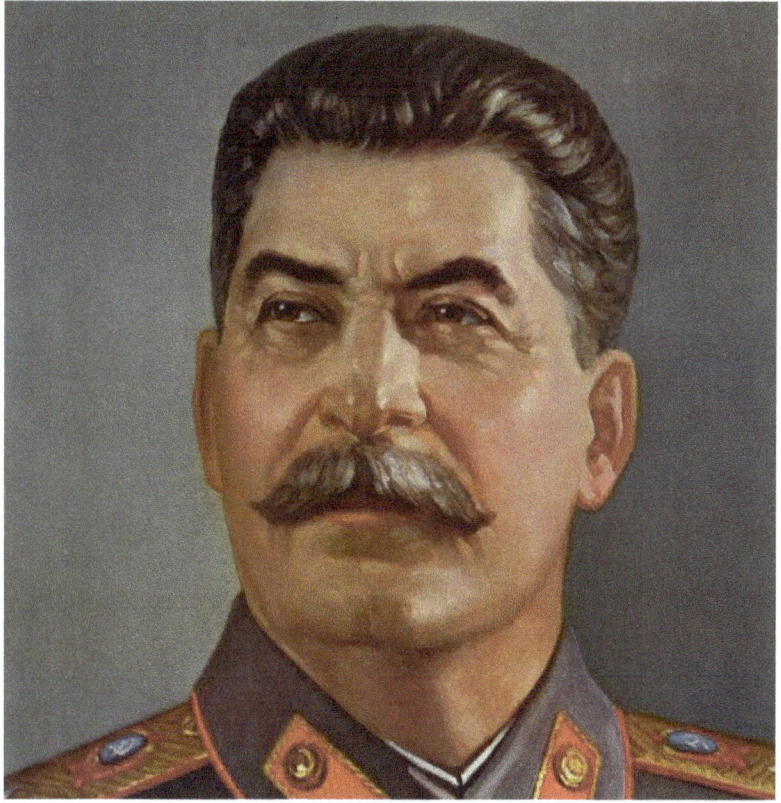

Josef Stalin, Public Domain

He did not hesitate to answer the call of nature and defecate openly in front of his entourage when a toilet was not readily available on a trip to the countryside. Apparently he drew the line of personal decency at farting. Stalin had a profound phobia of farting in public. When attending meetings, he would always have two water glasses in front of him that he would clink together repeatedly to mask the sound of his emanations.

Famous Quotations:

"A single death is a tragedy; a million deaths is a statistic."
"Those who vote decide nothing. Those who count the vote decide everything."
"Ideas are far more powerful than guns. We don't let our people have guns. Why should we let them have ideas?"
"Education is a weapon, whose effect depends on who holds it in his hands and at whom it is aimed."
"It is not heroes that make history, but history that makes heroes."
"This creature softened my heart of stone. She died and with her died my last warm feelings for humanity."
"When there's a person, there's a problem. When there's no person, there's no problem.

Sir Robert Hutchinson

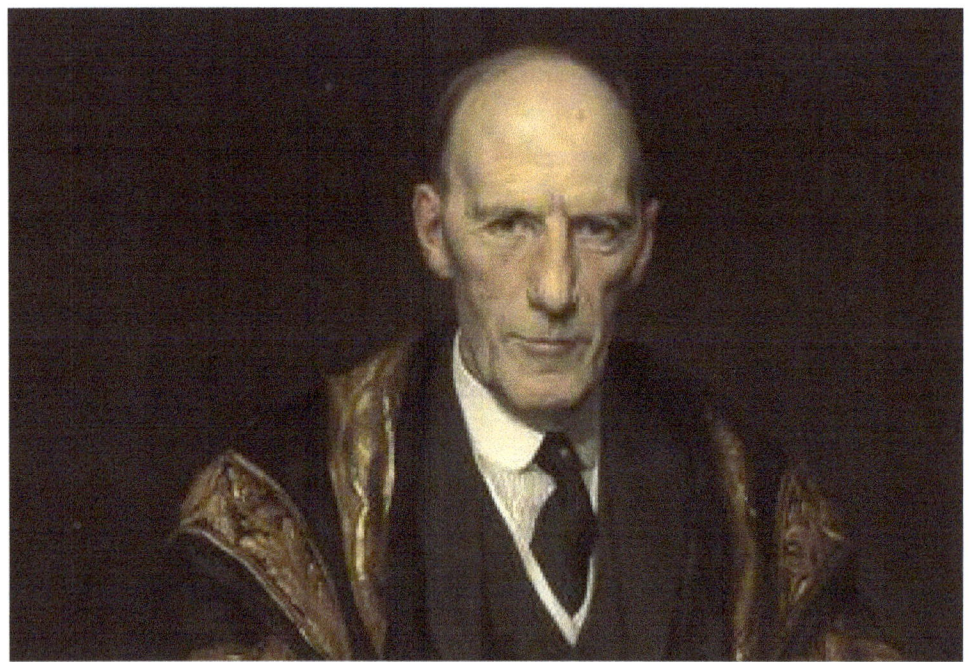

Sir Robert Grieve Hutchinson Accessed at www.bbc.co.uk 1938, Royal College of Physicians, London
Artist Herbert James Gunn

Sir Robert Grieve Hutchinson (1871-1960) was a Scottish physician, pediatrician, radiologist and philosopher. He was the editor of *Food and the Principles of Dietetics* and served as President of the Royal School of Medicine and the Royal College of Physicians. He was consultant pediatrician at the Great Ormond Street Hospital for Sick Children, which was the beneficiary of all royalties from J.M. Barrie's classic tale *Peter Pan.*

"Vegetarianism is harmless enough, though it is apt to fill a man with wind and self-righteousness."

Famous Quotation:

"From inability to let well alone;
from too much zeal for the new and contempt for what is old;
from putting knowledge before wisdom, science before art, and cleverness before common sense;
from treating patients as cases;
and from making the cure of the disease more grievous than the endurance of the same,
Good Lord, deliver us."

Charles de Gaulle

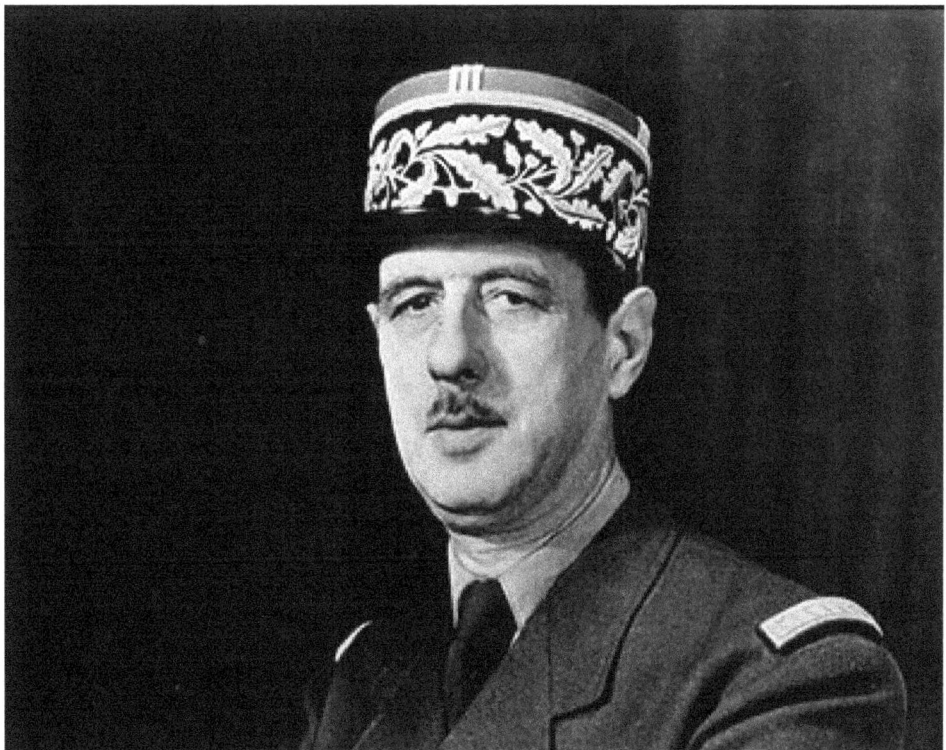

A WWII photo portrait of General Charles de Gaulle of the Free French Forces and first president of the Fifth Republic serving from 1959 to 1969. Library of Congress Public Domain

Charles André Joseph Marie de Gaulle (1890 – 1970) French general, statesman, president, and gourmand, Charles de Gaulle blamed his farts on a predilection for dishes prepared from offal.

Famous Quotations:

"How can you govern a country which has 246 varieties of cheese?"
"The better I get to know men, the more I find myself loving dogs."
"Silence is the ultimate weapon of power."
"A man of character finds a special attractiveness in difficulty, since it is only by coming to grips with difficulty that he can realize his potentialities."
"The cemeteries of the world are full of indispensable men."
"Don't ask me who's influenced me. A lion is made up of the lambs he's digested, and I've been reading all my life."
"I have come to the conclusion that politics are too serious a matter to be left to the politicians."
"Where there is a will, there is a way.."
"Patriotism is when love of your own people comes first; nationalism, when hate for people other than your own comes first."
"You'll live. Only the best get killed."
"Since a politician never believes what he says, he is surprised when others believe him."
"Nothing great will ever be achieved without great men, and men are great only if they are determined to be so."

Lyndon Baines Johnson

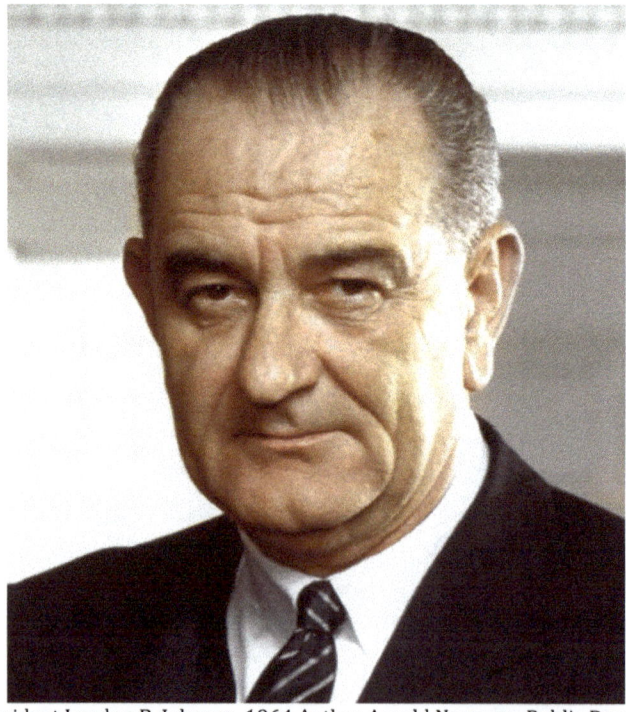

President Lyndon B. Johnson, 1964 Author Arnold Newman, Public Domain

Lyndon Baines Johnson (1908 – 1973) was the 36th President of the United States. He was of the outspoken opinion that U.S. Representative and future U.S. President Gerald Ford was not a very bright man. He used the memorable expression that his opinion was that Ford was so dumb that he could not chew gum and fart at the same time.

President Johnson was also known for his at times crude bathroom behavior, which he used to intimidate aides. He would often insist on subordinates continuing conversations with him, while he was seated on the toilet having a bowel movement and farting.

Famous Quotations:

"Yesterday is not ours to recover, but tomorrow is ours to win or lose."
"Books and ideas are the most effective weapons against intolerance and ignorance."
"We can draw lessons from the past, but we cannot live in it."
"I may not know much, but I know chicken shit from chicken salad."
"While you're saving your face, you're losing your ass."
"The noblest search is the search for excellence"
"Until justice is blind to color, until education is unaware of race, until opportunity is unconcerned with the color of men's skins, emancipation will be a proclamation but not a fact."

Ronald Reagan

Ronald Wilson Reagan (1911 – 2004) was the fortieth President of the United Sates. I heard an apocryphal story from a normally reliable source that served in a high position in the administration of former president Ronald Reagan. Then again the source was a politician, which should automatically double the suspicion that this story was just the continued passage of excessive hot air.

Her Majesty, Queen Elizabeth II was visiting the presidential ranch, Rancho Cielo, in the Santa Ynez Mountains of California. The ranch is at a high elevation (Rancho Cielo is Spanish for Sky Ranch) and as both the president and queen are horse aficionados they went for a ride on the ranch trails.

At higher altitude the atmospheric pressure is less than at sea level and thus the volume of gasses expands (Boyle's Law). The horse's intestinal tracts likewise experienced expanding gasses and being natural animals they release it at will, even if they are in the presence of a Royal Queen and President.

Along the trail the Queen's horse in particular became increasingly flatulent with noisy and pungent emissions. The smell became unbearable and the Queen said to Mr. Reagan. "Mr. President I really must apologize for the terrible aroma."

Some observers thought that perhaps President Reagans Alzheimer Disease was beginning to take hold, but much more likely it was his quick wit that rose to the occasion. Mr. Regan responded, "Your Majesty, you needn't have apologized at all. In fact, if you hadn't said anything, I would have thought it was the horses!"

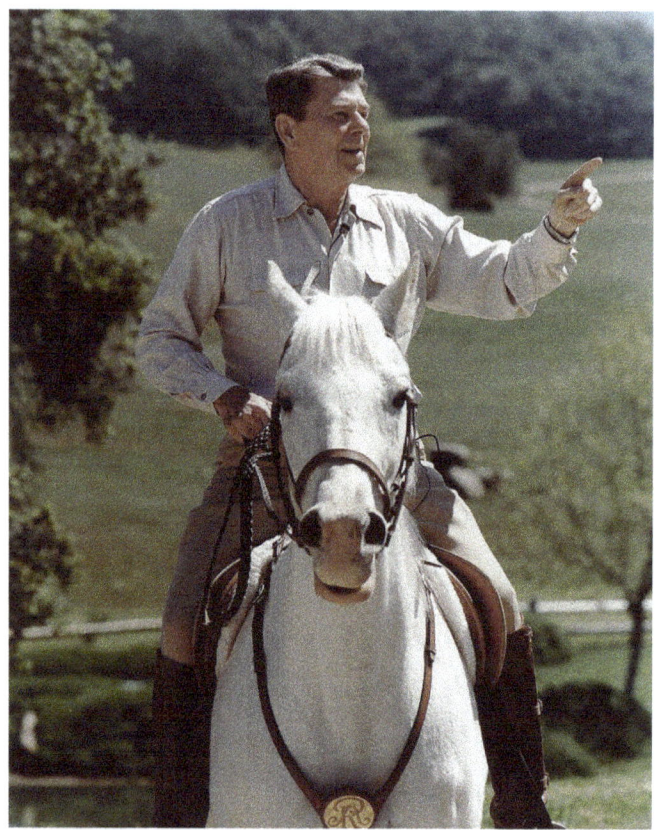

US President Ronald Reagan riding a white horse. 2004 Pete Souza official White House photographer Public Domain

Another story about President Reagan that he shared had to do with a secret service agent who was in a meeting room where the president and some advisors were to gather later in the day. Bowls of cashew nuts were on the table and the agent was helping himself to the hospitality with a cashew in his palm when the president walked in unexpectedly. The agent quickly palmed the evidence and kept his arms behind his back.

Apparently the President had gotten a quick glance at the agent's palm before it was quickly clenched and hidden from view. Mr. Reagan in a very supportive voice said to the agent that he needn't be embarrassed; he has to wear one too. The agent gratefully replied "Thank you, Mr. President" and promptly put the cashew in his ear as if it were the hearing aid the president thought he saw.

Famous Quotations:

"Government is like a baby: an alimentary canal with a big appetite at one end and no sense of responsibility at the other."
"The greatest leader is not necessarily the one who does the greatest things. He is the one that gets the people to do the greatest things."
"There is no limit to the amount of good you can do if you don't care who gets the credit."
"How do you tell a Communist? Well, it's someone who reads Marx and Lenin. And how do you tell an anti-Communist? It's someone who understands Marx and Lenin."
"Politics is not a bad profession. If you succeed there are many rewards, if you disgrace yourself you can always write a book."
"I've heard that hard work never killed anyone, but I say why take the chance?"
"It has been said that politics is the second oldest profession. I have learned that it bears a striking resemblance to the first."
"When you can't make them see the light, make them feel the heat."
"It isn't so much that liberals are ignorant. It's just that they know so many things that aren't so."
"Above all, we must realize that no arsenal, or no weapon in the arsenals of the world, is so formidable as the will and moral courage of free men and women."
"Surround yourself with great people; delegate authority; get out of the way"
"Never let the things you can't do, stop you from doing what you can."
"Let me speak plainly: The United States of America is and must remain a nation of openness to people of all beliefs. Our very unity has been strengthened by this pluralism. That's how we began; this is how we must always be. The ideals of our country leave no room whatsoever for intolerance, anti-Semitism, or bigotry of any kind -- none. The unique thing about America is a wall in our Constitution separating church and state. It guarantees there will never be a state religion in this land, but at the same time it makes sure that every single American is free to choose and practice his or her religious beliefs or to choose no religion at all. Their rights shall not be questioned or violated by the state.
"Peace is not absence of conflict, it is the ability to handle conflict by peaceful means."
"I was not a great communicator, but I communicated great things."
"The only thing necessary for the triumph of evil, is for good men to do nothing"

H.M. Queen Elizabeth II & H.R.H. Prince Philip

Queen Elizabeth II Alexandra Mary (1926 -) is the constitutional monarch of Great Britain. Prince Philip, (1921 -) Duke of Edinburgh, was born Prince Philip of Greece and Denmark.

As the prince consort and husband of Queen Elizabeth II he is the oldest and longest serving spouse of a reigning British monarch. He is also the oldest-ever male member of the British royal family. As the series of photographs above document with astonishing clarity, he may also now be officially proclaimed a royal 'Old Fart'.

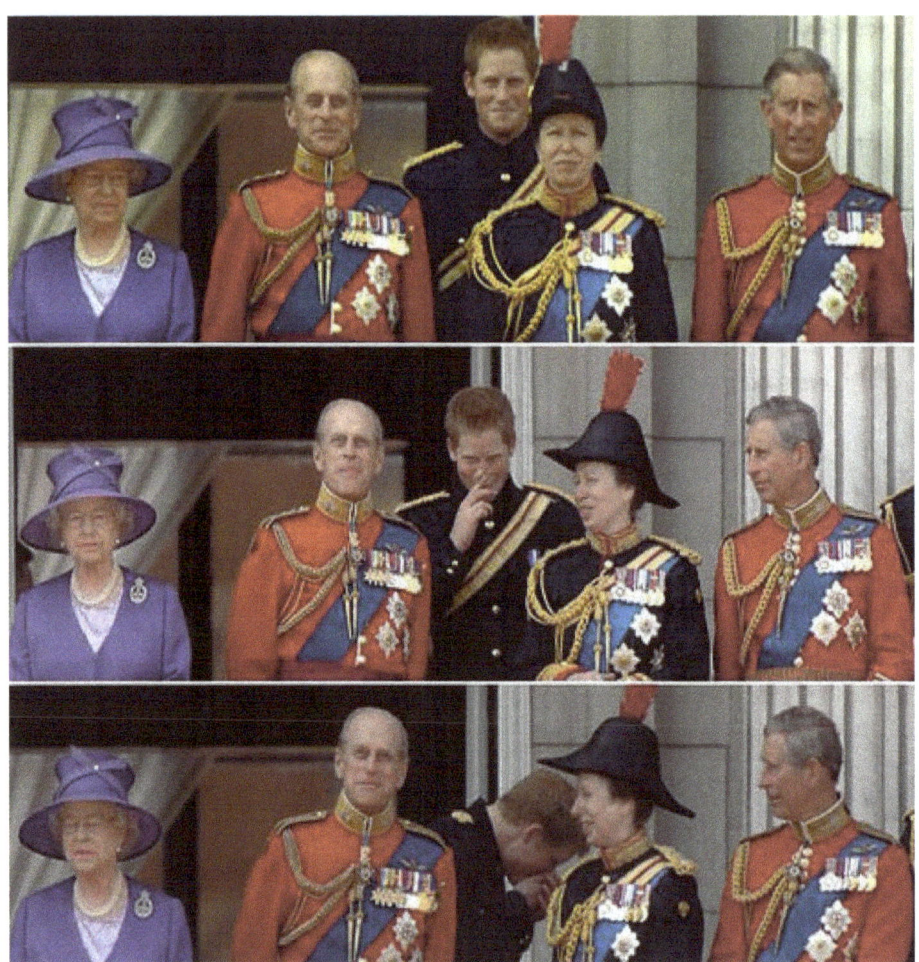

A royal fart at a royal wedding.

Queen Elizabeth is known to have a healthy sense of humor. During the Second World War she served in her country's military as a driver. Her military grade driving skills over rough roads at her Scottish country estate of Balmoral became the source of a humorous story she shared with Sir Shepard Cowper-Coles, the United Kingdom Ambassador to Saudi Arabia.

After lunch, the Queen had asked her royal guest, Crown Prince Abdullah, the future King of Saudi Arabia, whether he would like a tour of the estate. Prompted by his foreign minister the urbane Prince Saud, an initially hesitant Abdullah had agreed. The royal Land Rovers were drawn up in front of the castle. As instructed, the Crown Prince climbed into the front seat of the front Land Rover, his interpreter in the seat behind.

To his surprise, the Queen climbed into the driving seat, turned the ignition and drove off. Women are not — yet — allowed to drive in Saudi Arabia, and Abdullah was not used to being driven by a woman, let alone a queen.

His nervousness only increased as the Queen, an Army driver in wartime, accelerated the Land Rover along the narrow Scottish estate roads, talking all the time. Through his interpreter, the Crown Prince implored the Queen to slow down and concentrate on the road ahead.

Famous Quotation:

Grief is the price we pay for love.

George W. Bush

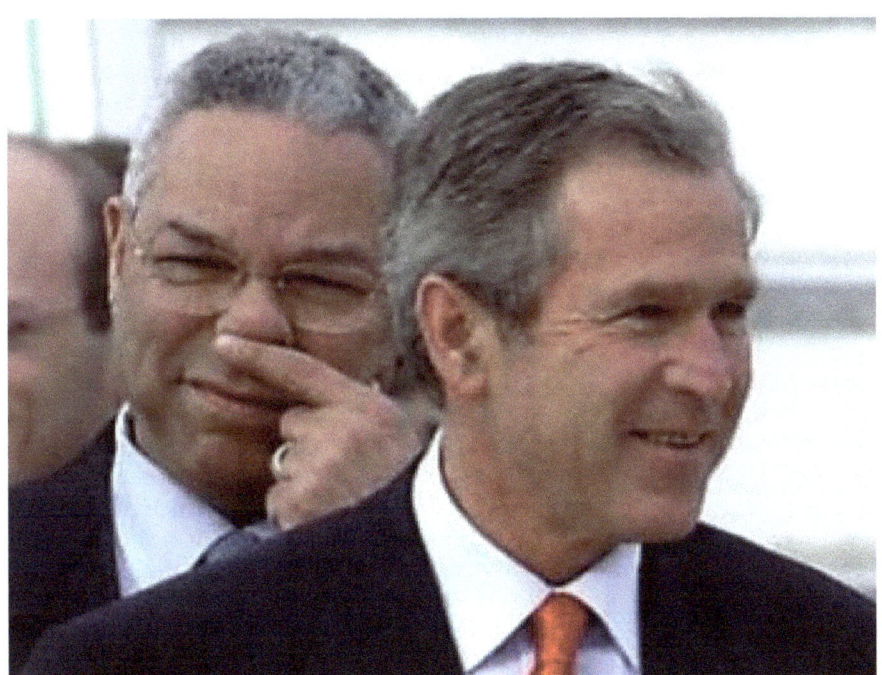

George W. Bush and U.S. Secretary of State Colin Powell. Public Domain

George Walker Bush (1946 -) was the 43rd President of the United States. He has a well-reported fondness for bathroom humor and fart jokes. As the photograph below illustrates he may be releasing more than just fart joke.

The photograph also brings to mind the term 'fart catcher'. This was a commonly used but derisive term for a valet or footman used to walking behind his master or mistress, or if on a horse and carriage, riding behind the horse.

Famous Quotations:

"They misunderestimated me."
"In my sentences I go where no man has gone before."
"We will not tire, we will not falter, and we will not fail."
"Our enemies are innovative and resourceful, and so are we. They never stop thinking about new ways to harm our country and our people, and neither do we."
"I think we agree, the past is over. "
"It will take time to restore chaos"
"Freedom is not our gift to the world it is God's gift to humanity."
"The thing that's wrong with the French is that they don't have a word for entrepreneur"
"To those of you who received honors, awards , and distinctions, I say, well done. And to the C students I say, you, too, can be president of the United States."
"I have opinions of my own, strong opinions, but I don't always agree with them."
"Recognizing and confronting our history is important. Transcending our history is essential. We are not limited by what we have done, or what we have left undone. We are limited only by what we are willing to do."

Muammar Gaddafi

Muammar Gaddafi (c. 1942 – 2011) was a revolutionary, politician, and de facto dictator of the country of Libya for forty-two years. He was eccentric, controversial, and maintained the rank of Colonel to bolster his image as a humble revolutionary. US President Reagan described him as an international pariah and the mad dog of the Middle East.

Colonel Gaddafi used to serve visiting foreign dignitaries camel milk for his own amusement. He knew that it caused explosive diarrhea and flatulence in those exposed to the product for the first time. When traveling abroad, he would set up a traditional Bedouin tent encampment for himself and his entourage. He always brought his herd of lactating camels with him to ensure he had access to a supply of fresh camel milk. As a result of all the nourishing camel's milk he drank, Muammar Gaddafi was famously flatulent.

At a summit meeting Colonel Gaddafi sat with British Prime Minister Tony Blair in the dictator's tent. He repeatedly invited Blair to try a glass of camel's milk, a Bedouin specialty. Subsequent news reports provided background color commentary to their interaction. "Don't touch it," Blair's interpreter insisted. Blair duly resisted. Afterwards, he asked the interpreter: "What's wrong with the camel's milk?" The interpreter replied: "If you've not had it before, you get the runs in five minutes and fart like a trumpet - and Gaddafi knows it."

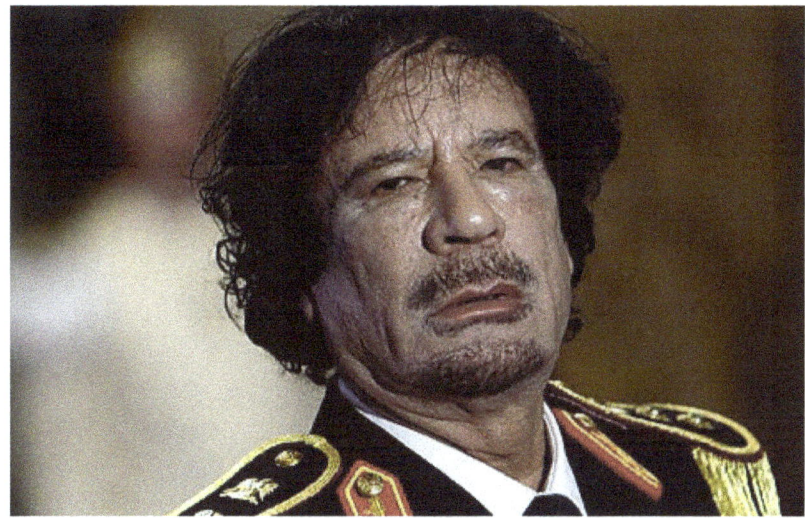
Muammar Gaddafi, Public Domain

Famous Quotations:

"There is no state with a democracy except Libya on the whole planet."
"Democracy means permanent rule"
"No representation of the people-representation is a falsehood. The mere existence of parliaments underlies the absence of the people, for democracy can only exist with the presence of the people and not in the presence of representatives of the people."
"A woman has a right to run for election whether she is male or female"
"Women, like men, are human beings. Women are different from men in form because they are females, just as all females in the kingdom of plants and animals differ from the male of their species"
"I cannot recognize either the Palestinian state or the Israeli state. The Palestinians are idiots and the Israelis are idiots."
"Another grave historical error is for several religions to remain in existence after Muhammad."
"Labor in return for wages is virtually the same as enslaving a human being."
"All African nations look up to Libya, all the rulers of the world look up to Libya. Protesters are serving the devil."
"If a community of people wears white on a mournful occasion and another dresses in black, then one community would like white and dislike black and the other would like black and dislike white. Moreover, this attitude leaves a physical effect on the cells as well as on the genes in the body."

H.H. the 14th Dalai Lama of Tibet

His Holiness the 14th Dalai Lama of Tibet is known for his robust appreciation for humor and happiness in life. With frequent lectures and appearances around the world he is an experienced air traveler. In an appearance in 2013 in Adelaide Australia he relates how he has been bothered by digestive gas while at high altitude.

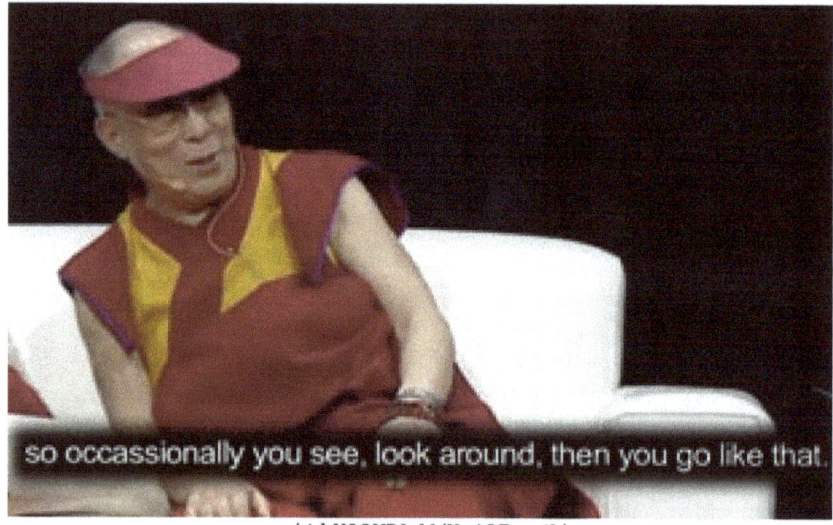

m/-i-hH9OVDIoM/Uo4O7yvqjI/

He describes how he tries to be discrete as he relives himself of this excess gas. "When in aeroplane, sometimes this gas problem comes. Then, you see, it is difficult to let out. So, occasionally, you see, look around, then you go like that." Perhaps this brings a new meaning to enlightenment, as well as to how yogis developed the ability to levitate.

Famous Quotations:

"Love is the absence of judgment."
"My religion is very simple. My religion is kindness."
"People take different roads seeking fulfillment and happiness. Just because they're not on your road doesn't mean they've gotten lost."
"This is my simple religion. No need for temples. No need for complicated philosophy. Your own mind, your own heart is the temple. Your philosophy is simple kindness."
"If you want others to be happy, practice compassion. If you want to be happy, practice compassion."
"Remember that sometimes not getting what you want is a wonderful stroke of luck."
 "Sleep is the best meditation."
"Peace does not mean an absence of conflicts; differences will always be there. Peace means solving these differences through peaceful means; through dialogue, education, knowledge; and through humane ways."

"Irrespective of whether we are believers or agnostics, whether we believe in God or karma, moral ethics is a code which everyone is able to pursue."
"If scientific analysis were conclusively to demonstrate certain claims in Buddhism to be false, then we must accept the findings of science and abandon those claims."
"Be kind whenever possible. It is always possible."
"All suffering is caused by ignorance. People inflict pain on others in the selfish pursuit of their own happiness or satisfaction"
"Love and compassion are necessities, not luxuries. Without them, humanity cannot survive."
"Know the rules well, so you can break them effectively."
"We can never obtain peace in the outer world until we make peace with ourselves."
"Our prime purpose in this life is to help others. And if you can't help them, at least don't hurt them."
"If a problem is fixable, if a situation is such that you can do something about it, then there is no need to worry. If it's not fixable, then there is no help in worrying. There is no benefit in worrying whatsoever."

"Man surprised me most about humanity. Because he sacrifices his health in order to make money. Then he sacrifices money to recuperate his health. And then he is so anxious about the future that he does not enjoy the present; the result being that he does not live in the present or the future; he lives as if he is never going to die, and then dies having never really lived."

Global Warming

Global warming due to greenhouse gas production from human activity is mainly due to deforestation, the combustion of fossil fuels, livestock enteric fermentation and manure management, and landfill emissions. In terms of biomass bacteria would be the main contributors to global warming by their methane production.

Other contenders nominated have been termites, which have over 2000 species and are prolific methane producers (initial reports suggested that they produce 40% of global methane), livestock such as cows, sheep, and pigs, and lastly dinosaurs, which are no longer around to defend their reputations.

A ruminant (Latin *ruminare* - to chew over again) is a mammal that digests plants in a multi compartment stomach through bacterial fermentation. It regurgitates the semi-digested mass, called cud, and chews it again and repeats the swallow. The process of rechewing the cud is called "ruminating". There are about 150 species of ruminants, which include both domestic and wild species. Ruminating mammals include cattle, goats, sheep, giraffes, yaks, deer, camels, llamas, and antelope.

Artsy Fartsy: Cultural History of the Fart Volume One

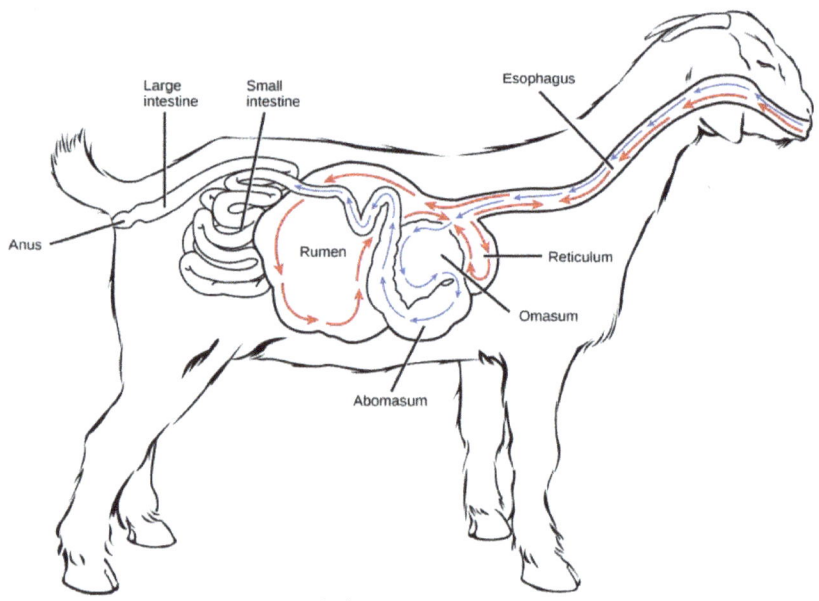

www.rice.edu/ Creative Commons License

FLATULENCE TAX

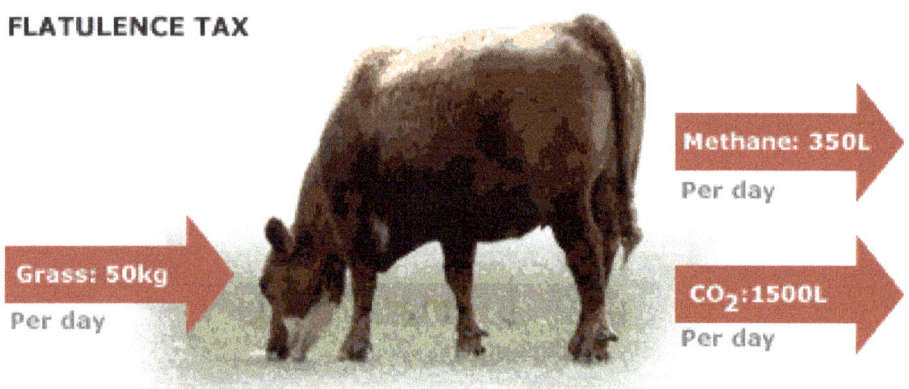

	COW	SHEEP
Example herd size	500	3,000
Methane produced*	63,875,000	21,900,000
CO2 produced*	273,750,000	82,125,000
Tax per litre	$0.046	$0.0003
Tax per farmer	$300	$300

*- Litres per year

In spite of it being labeled as a flatulence tax, the predominant source of global warming from ruminants comes from fermentation in their multi compartment stomachs. It should really be called a burping and belching tax, but that is not as newsworthy.

Ruminant bacterial fermentation is a significant contributor to global methane production, which is over twenty times as potent a greenhouse gas as carbon dioxide. To incentivize efforts to reduce livestock methane production a number of countries have proposed taxes on the release of greenhouse gasses.

The public debate generated by the proposed tax added to global warming with media interviews, editorials, and vocal bovine protests as illustrated below. Farmers have complained loudly that the whole tax concept stinks and should be expelled promptly from any further consideration.

University of Alberta, Canada, Professor Stephen Moore is examining the genes from ruminant stomachs with the goal of developing a cow breed which burps less to reduce methane in the greenhouse gases responsible for global warming. His work was published in 2009 in the Journal of Animal Science.

A different approach is being undertaken by Professor of Animal Nutrition Winfried Drochner at the University of Hohenheim, Stuttgart, Germany. A fist-sized plant-based pill bolus combined with a special diet and strict feeding times reduces the methane produced by cows. "Our aim is to increase the wellbeing of the cow, to reduce the greenhouse gases produced and to increase agricultural production all at once. It is an effective way of fighting global warming. We could use the energy to boost the cow's metabolism, the fist-sized tablets mean that microbiotic substances can slowly dissolve in the cow's stomach over several months," said Prof Drochner.

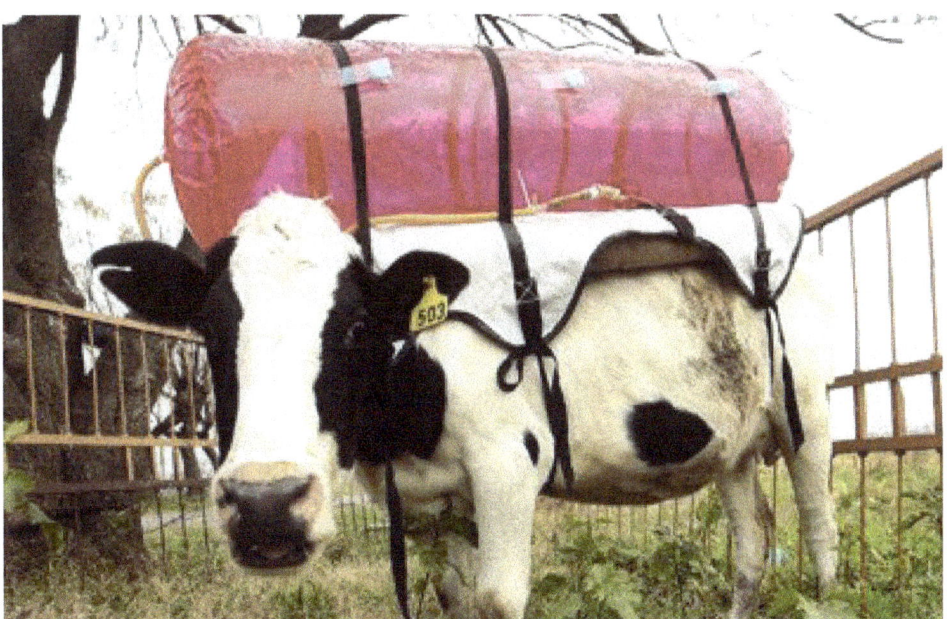

Science at work measuring bovine intestinal gas production. Public Domain.

Another method being used to reduce methane emissions is reducing the grass and low efficiency foods the livestock are receiving that require excessive fermentation. Replacing the feed with a diet higher in energy and rich in edible oils can reduce methane production by up to twenty-five percent.

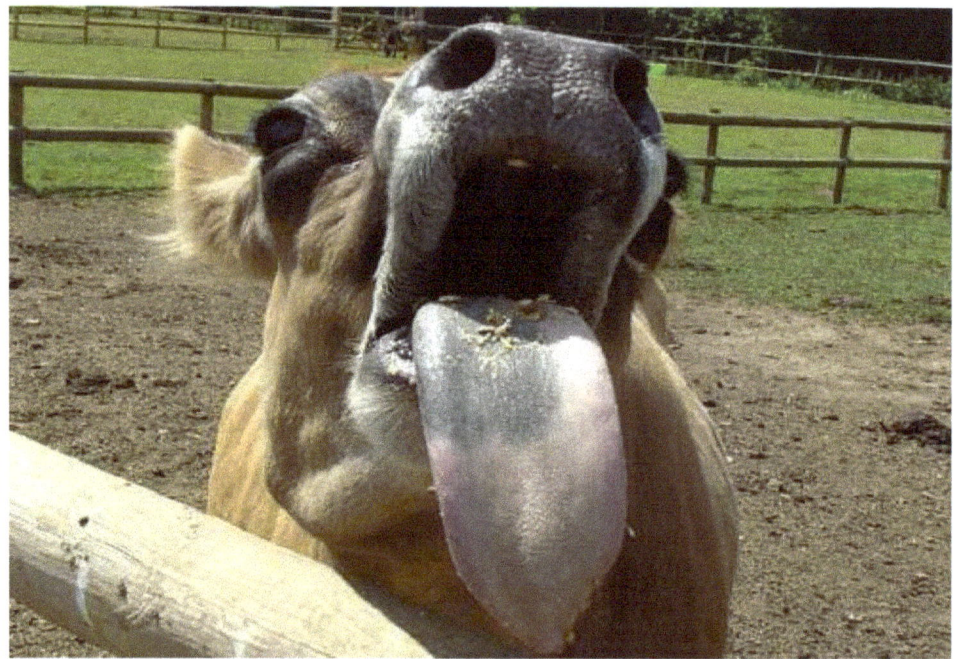
It is the burps and belches from the multi compartment ruminant stomach that is the primary source of methane. Public Domain

New Hampshire-based Stonyfield Farm reduced emissions from their cows an average of twelve percent by adding alfalfa, flax or hemp to livestock feed. 'If every U.S. dairy farmer reduced emissions by twelve percent it would be equal to about half a million cars being taken off the road,' said Nancy Hirshberg, vice president of Stonyfield's Natural Resources department.

It took extensive scientific experimentation to collect the intestinal gasses of herds of cattle before it was discovered that the methane production was coming from the other end of the cows and other ruminants. It is the burps and belches from the multi compartment ruminant stomach that is the primary source of methane.

The Great Chicago Fire which destroyed the city in 1871 has traditionally been blamed on Mrs. O'Leary's cow kicking over a kerosene lamp. With the large volume of methane produced it is just as likely to have been caused by her cow farting and belching,. But that would not have been an acceptable cause in Victorian times.

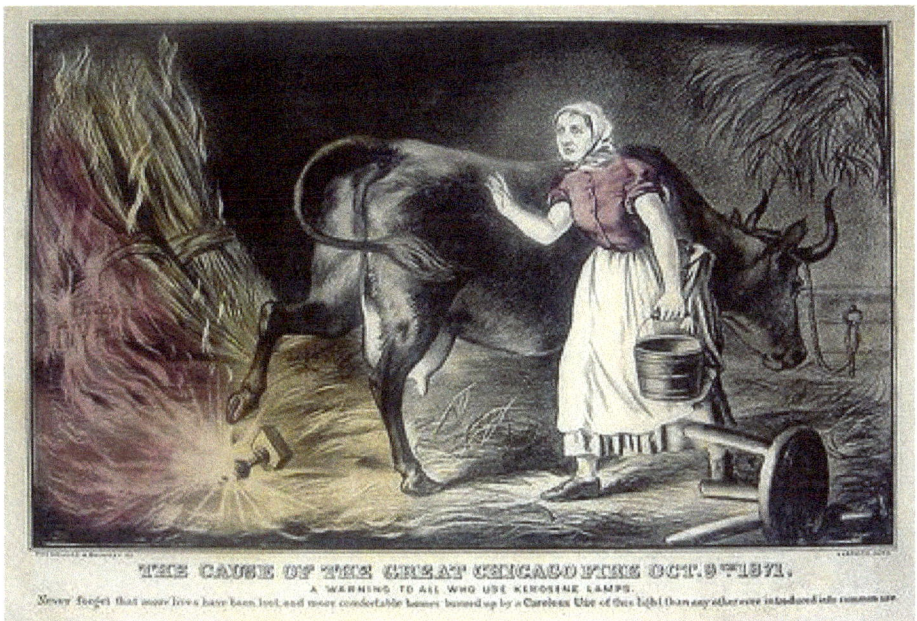
Public Domain

Kangaroos are herbivores and as marsupial their burps and farts contain little or no methane, a potent greenhouse gas. It appears that the reduced methane emissions are due to the microbes in the kangaroos' gut flora. Australian researchers hope that introducing a similar gut flora to other methane producing herbivores such as cattle and sheep will contribute to a reduction in greenhouse gasses and the resultant global warming. Methane can cause about 20 times as much atmospheric warming as an equivalent volume of carbon dioxide.

Kangaroos, like cattle and sheep, are ruminants that rechew their cud with the assistance of the gut flora to digest the and metabolize their cellulose based grazing diet. In the foregut the meal is broken down by fermentation with carbon dioxide and hydrogen released. In cows and other ruminants, microbes called methanogens transform these gases into methane. But in the kangaroos' guts the same hydrogen and carbon dioxide may be utilized by bacteria called acetogens to produce acetate, a volatile fatty acid.

These microbes compete with methanogens to use the carbon dioxide and hydrogen, so the more acetogens the less methane production. The odds are in generally in favor of methanogens, since the process of methane production is generally more energy efficient than producing acetate. One of the acetogen microbes, *Blautia coccoides*, live in cows as well as in kangaroos. Further research is being undertaken to understand why the organism is more successful in competing with the methanogens in kangaroos than in other herbivores.

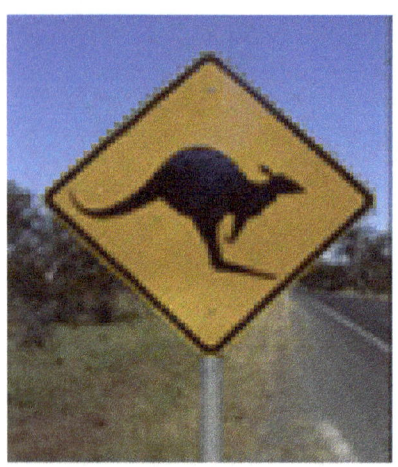

Kangaroo Farts Could Help Curb Warming

Secret to methane-free gas could be transferred to cattle and sheep

img1-azcdn.newser.com

Carbon dioxide, methane, nitrous oxide, and three groups of fluorinated gases (sulfur hexafluoride, hydro fluorocarbons , and per fluorocarbons) are the major greenhouse gases impacted by human activity. These are regulated under the Kyoto Protocol an international treaty that was adopted in 2005.

Nitrogen dioxide (NO2) warms the atmosphere three hundred and ten times more than carbon dioxide, and methane twenty-one times more than carbon dioxide. Although CFCs are greenhouse gases, regulations were initiated because CFCs' cause ozone depletion, not because of their contribution to global warming. Ozone depletion itself has a relatively minor effect on greenhouse warming.

Dinosaurs are no longer around to defend themselves and have been accused of contributing to global warming. We do not know if they were ruminants and contributed by belching up gasses as well, but there should be no doubt that they were big time farters. Their nickname "thunder lizards" may have more to do with their farts than their footsteps.

The hulking sauropods were widespread about 150 million years ago, and methane-producing microbes aided the sauropods' digestion by fermenting their plant food. Dave Wilkinson of Liverpool John Moores University, Graeme Ruxton from the University of Saint Andrews, and methane expert Euan Nisbet at the University of London studied the implications. Wilkinson, Ruxton, and Nisbet calculated global methane emissions from sauropods to have been approximately 520 million tons per year. By comparison modern livestock ruminant animals produce methane emission of up to 100 million tons per year.

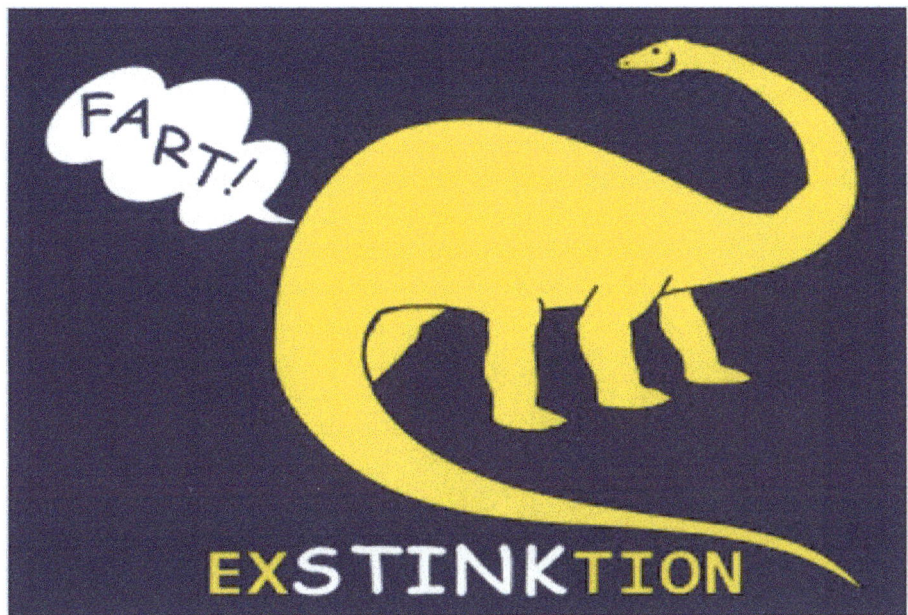

www.astropt.org Creative Commons License

"A simple mathematical model suggests that the microbes living in sauropod dinosaurs may have produced enough methane to have an important effect on the Mesozoic climate. Indeed, our calculations suggest that these dinosaurs could have produced more methane than all modern sources -- both natural and man-made -- put together. Clearly, trying to estimate this for animals that are unlike anything living has to be a bit of an educated guess," Wilkinson said.

Continued in Volume Two

IX. Colloquialism, Idiom, & Synonym of Fart

The word fart is one of the oldest words in the English language. One of the most important dictionaries in the long history of the language is Samuel Johnson's *A Dictionary of the English Language* published in 1755. An important innovation in his dictionary was the use of quotations from literature to illustrate the usage of the word defined.

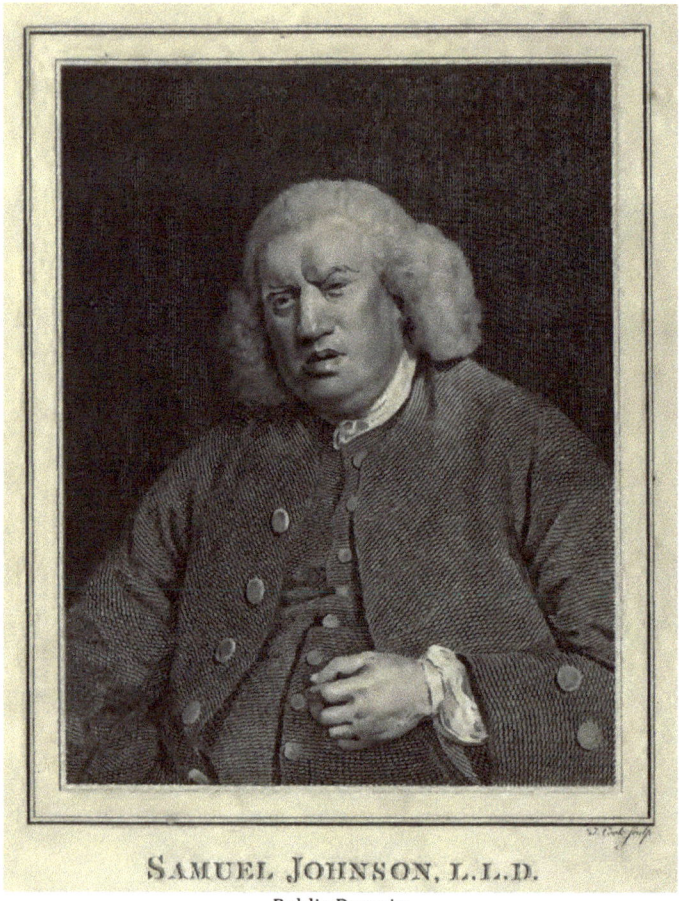

Public Domain

The word fart is proper English, and was in use for hundreds of years, before relatively recent polite and civil society considered it taboo. Without an alternative word, euphemisms were created and used. The number of terms that were synonymous with fart numbers in the many hundreds. The partial list that follows gives a good approximation of the wide variety of colorful alternatives.

The origins of these phrases, and their acceptance into the cultural lexicon, are often obscured. Sometimes new words are added simply by an author creatively using a newly invented word in a literary work. I am fond of a new word coined by David Gilmour, an entrepreneur and philanthropist. He described a word that combines the sense of anticipation and subsequent disappointment, when the experience is not as satisfying as expected. The word he crated 'anticipointment' is a portmanteau that should stand the test of time.

I am tempted to add to new words to the lexicon as well. I am using the author's prerogative to place the words in print below, and although I have not heard them elsewhere before someone may well have created them before me. The first word is fartigenic, or its alternative, fartogenic. Fartigenic is a portmanteau combining the word fart with the Latin root suffix -genic of genesis and creation fame. The word describes a substance, which induces the creation of a fart. Refried beans and chili con carne would be good examples of fartigenic foods.

My second word creation choice would be related to the common phrase stomach flu when used to describe a viral gastroenteritis with diarrhea and farting. We often use the term flu when describing a viral illness even though in is not a true influenza virus. I am taking poetic liberty to borrow the influenza root word to describe a stomach flu as 'inflatuenza'.

My third and final word would be an alternative word for bloating or distention. As one could consider this condition to be caused by the retention and delay of the necessary intestinal gas passage, I suggest the word 'gastipated'. Okay, so maybe that word will not stand the test of time, and I should cease my word mining activities while I still have you as a reader.

What follows are the colloquialisms, idioms, and synonyms, that for better or for worse, are part of the lexicon.

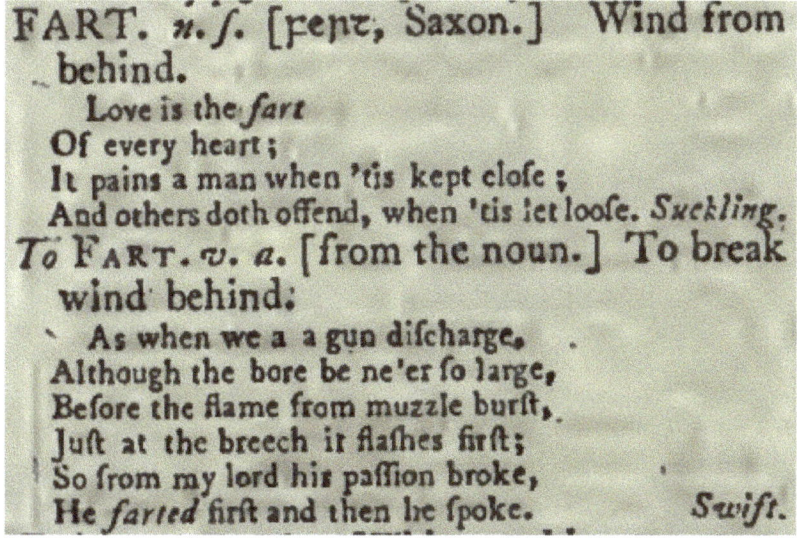
Public Domain

A bit more choke and you would have started – an Australian phrase often addressed to the person responsible for an audible fart
Afflatus – Although it contains the word flatus this word has nothing to do with a fart. Flatus is Latin for a blowing, breathing, or a wind. Afflatus is a word first used by Cicero in his volume *De Natura Deorum* (*The Nature of the Gods*). In his book it is used as a phrase for a sudden rush of unexpected breath, a fresh inspiration. The word inspiration is derived from inspire, to breath as well as to have a creative thought or new idea. Afflatus thus can mean a divine inspiration. The only way to associate it with a fart is to consider it to be the exact opposite of a brain fart.
After thunder comes the rain – Phrase used when fart is passed just before urinating.
Air bagel – Fart
Air biscuit – Fart
Anal acoustics - Fart
Anal ahem - Fart
Anal audio - Fart
Anal salute - Fart
Anal volcano - Fart
Aqua fart - An underwater fart bubble, usually seen in the bathtub or swimming pool. The only way to clearly see an otherwise invisible fart.
Arse blast - Fart
Artsy Fartsy – Presented as art and culture but just as likely to be seen as pretentious, eccentric, eclectic, and unworthy of sophisticated cultural approval.
As much chance as a fart in a thunderstorm, windstorm, blizzard, hurricane, tornado, gale, etcetera - Means having no chance at all.
Ass blaster - Fart
Ass biscuit - Fart
Ass thunder - Fart
Ass whistle - Fart
Brain fart – Mental lapse, which usually results in an error while doing a repetitive activity.
Backdoor breeze - Fart
Backfire - Fart
Barking spiders - Fart
Bean blower - Fart
Blast off - Fart
Blowing a Raspberry (or Strawberry) – Imitating the sound of a fart by exhaling through pursed lips, usually as a sign of derision. Also known as a Bronx cheer.
Blowing the butt bugle - Fart
Blowing you a kiss - Fart
Bomber - Fart
Bottom blast - Fart
Bottom burp - Fart
Break wind - Fart

Artsy Fartsy: Cultural History of the Fart Volume One

Breath of fresh air - Fart
Bronx cheer - Imitating the sound of a fart by exhaling through pursed lips, usually as a sign of derision. Also known as a Blowing a Raspberry or Strawberry.
Brown horn brass choir - Fart
Brown thunder - Fart
Bun shaker - Fart
Burnin' rubber - Fart
Buster - Fart
Busting ass - Fart
Butt bleat - Fart
Butt burp - Fart
Butt percussion - Fart
Butt trumpet - Fart
Butt tuba - Fart
Buttock bassoon - Fart
Cheek flapper - Fart
Cheesin' - Fart
Colonic calliope - Fart
Crack a rat - Fart
Crack one off - Fart
Crack splitters - Fart
Crop dusting - Farting while passing seated bystanders
Crowd splitter - Fart
Cut a stinker - Fart
Cut loose - Fart
Cut the cheese - Fart
Cut the wind - Fart
Death breath - Fart
Deflate - Fart
Drop a barking spider - Fart
Drop a bomb - Fart
Drop ass - Fart
Dutch oven – Farting under the blankets while in bed, then covering up your bedmate to share the aroma.
Empty my tank - Fart
Eproctophilia – A fart fetish, the receiving of sexual pleasure and arousal from the fart of another. The author James Joyce (see separate entry) describes this fetish in letters published after his death.
Exploding bottom - Fart
Exterminate - Fart
Farst – Descriptive of a fast fart

Fart – (Foreign languages) – Unrelated to the English usage of the word, in the German and Scandinavian languages the word means speed, often used in speeding or speed control zones signs. in Danish a *fartcertifikate* means a trade certificate. In Norwegian a *fart plan* means a schedule. The Norwegian phrase *stå*

Artsy Fartsy: Cultural History of the Fart Volume One

på fartin pronounced as stop-a –fartin means ready to leave. Likewise the phrase *farts måler* pronounced as fart smeller refers to a speedometer. In Swedish a speed bump is called a *farthinder*. *Fartlek* is speed training by running at alternate intervals of fast and slow paces.. Likewise if you travel on a Scandinavian marine vessel you may see the control of engine speed labeled as *half fart* and *full fart* for half speed and full speed respectively. Fart kontrol zones are speed zones. In Germany a similar word *fahrt* means a journey, trip, tour, or passage. It is often seen in signs that say e*infahrt* (sounds like in-fart) and *ausfahrt* (sounds like out-fart) denoting entrance and exit respectively. In Spanish and Portuguese *fart* means an excess of anything, especially a food. One of the richest deserts they offer is called a *farte*, which means a fruit tarte in Spain and usually a sugar almond or cream cake in Portugal. In Italy the word *farto* means mattress. In Hungarian *fartaj* means buttocks. In Poland if you want to buy a popular candy bar with a name that that means lucky you will be looking for a *Fart* bar.

Fartalito - Word for a small fart combining English and Spanish   (Spanglish)
Fartable farter – An individual who can fart on command
Fart about – Waste time on silly or unnecessary activities
Fart absorption ratio – Humorous descriptive of the quantity of farts that a material can absorb and retain before the trapped gas escapes. Usually used to describe furniture such as a chair, sofa, ottoman, cushions, mattress, but can also be applied to rugs, carpets, clothing, etcetera.
Fart ache – Descriptive of a fart so potent that exposure to the fumes gives a headache. May also be used to describe pain after farting with anorectal disease such as fissures, abscess, fistula, hemorrhoids, and after delivery or surgery.
Fartachoo – A fart and sneeze occurring simultaneously
Fartacious – Ability to produce copious farts, either by volume or frequency.
Fartacrite – An individual who is hypocritical about farts, considering the farts of others as objectionable while their own farts are perfectly acceptable.
Fart addict – One who is obsessed with farting, usually used to describe an individual who produces farts in prodigious frequency and quantity.
Fartage - (French) Waxing of cross-country skis, unrelated to fart.
Fart against thunder – The fart equivalent of urinating (pissing) into the wind.
Fartagious – Contagious farting, often noted in preadolescent males.
Fartaholic – An individual who is described as being addicted to farting, often used to describe a husband.
Fart alarm – When the need to fart is misinterpreted as the need to defecate. Also when a baby's diaper is changed assuming a bowel movement occurred, only to find the diaper is empty as it was just a fart.
Fartalicious – A particularly attractive fart, either by acoustics, aroma, or quantity. Also may be used as a sarcastic compliment denoting that the taste of a food or drink was offensive.
Fart amnesty – A zone where unhindered farting is allowed without criticism or limitation. The zone is usually defined by the significant other, and may be in a remote location and different time zone.
Fart and dart – An individual who release a fart and quickly departs to let others

experience their fart. Also known as fart and run.
Fart and flee – A practical joke, often executed spontaneously on releasing a fart in a crowded public place. The person immediately behind you is left standing in the aromatic wake of your fart, is assumed to be the culprit, and is the recipient of abhorrent glares from others.
Fart angels – Actively moving arms and legs in the same fashion as one makes snow angels by lying down in the snow. The activity is done in the standing mode to help circulate the air in the hope of dissipating the smell.
Fartanoid – A frantic sense of insecurity that an impending fart may allow the release of bowel contents.
Fartapalooza – A spasm of frequent, voluminous, and typically audacious farts over a short period of time. More often occurs following ingestion of a fart inducing meal, such as refried beans.
Fart app – An application for mobile phones and other electronic devices that reproduces sounds that imitate the various acoustic forms of the art of the fart.
Fart around – Waste time on silly or unnecessary activities
Fart arpeggio – A fart that changes tone at least twice so that three or more notes are produced during its course. A master of this technique was Joseph Pujol, known as Le Pétomane, during his performance career on the Moulin Rouge in Paris.
Fartarrhea – Similar to shart as a combination of shit and fart, but with diarrhea and fart. The fart often releases a mist of liquid feces, which soil the underwear or clothing if not released while on a toilet.
Fart arse – (British) To be stupid, farting or mucking around.
Fart art – Euphemism for abstract art appearance of soiling of underwear upon passing a particularly powerful fart that carried some organic fecal matter, mucus, or moisture. More common with a bout of dysentery or diarrhea.
Fart ass – Similar to smart-ass
Fart attack – Condition of pain related to intestinal gas, including intestinal gas in the pre-fart stage of bloating and distension. Play on words with similarity to heart attack, Unfortunately symptoms that suggest intestinal gas discomfort (fart attack) may actually be due to a heart condition (heart attack) and delay urgently needed medical care. In this situation a misdiagnosed fart/heart attack can be a true life threatening condition.
Fart baby – Descriptive term for abdominal bloating from intestinal gas, more noticeable in young thin women who develop visible distension that gives the impression of an early pregnancy.
Fart bag – A plastic or paper bag used to capture and seal in a fart, to be subsequently opened in the face of an unsuspecting victim.
Fart bellows – Farting under a blanket while in bed, and then trying to clear the fart by using the blanket as a bellow. The opposite of a Dutch oven, where the goal is to trap the fart under the blanket.
Fart blanche – To be given carte blanche to fart at will under the blanket or other locations.
Fart box – A euphemism for anus, rectum, and rectal cavity.

Fart brain – Used similarly to airhead, suggesting that farts rather than brains reside in the skull
Fart breath – Foul smelling breath
Fart bride – A woman who was very discrete about bodily functions, especially farts, before marriage, but loses all inhibitions after marriage.
Fart bubble – An underwater fart bubble, usually seen in the bathtub or swimming pool. The only way to clearly see an otherwise invisible fart.
Fart catcher – Nickname given to horsemen seated immediately behind the horses pulling a carriage. Also used to describe assistants and servants who walk a few paces behind their superior.
Fart buddy – A friend who is close enough that farting in their presence does not lead to any offense, and may contribute to an open farting atmosphere.
Fart burn – The burning rectal or anal sensation after extensive diarrhea and farting. Also may be experienced after eating hotly spiced foods.
Fart camouflage – Also known as fart camo. Making noise by an activity to hide the sound of a fart. The goal is to create a distraction to allow the noisy passage of a fart to go undetected. Using an air freshener, perfume, or other strong aroma may be used in an attempt to mask the smell. Opening windows and doors with the excuse that it is too warm is often used as a fart camouflage maneuver.
Fart candy – Candy that induces farting by having a high content of non-absorbable sugars. Dietetic candies often have this property.
Fart door - Colloquial term for anus.
Farter – A person who procrastinates by farting around. (British) Slang term for anus, also a sleeping bag which is warmed by farts.
Farterbox – (Irish) Slang for anus
Fartface – Facial expression that gives the impression that the wearer is smelling a noxious fart. Also slang for an idiot or stupid person.
Fart factory – Slang for anus, also to describe a frequent or voluminous farter.
Fart fetish – Formally known as eproctophilia, the receiving of sexual pleasure and arousal from the fart of another. The author James Joyce (see separate entry) describes this fetish in letters published after his death.
Farther, Farthest, Farthermost – These words denote greater distance from an object, an are unrelated to the word fart that is contained within their spelling. The only way they may be tied to the word fart is in vocabulary games like Scrabble, Boggle, and others where additional points may be gained by adding letters to a core word.
Fart higher than your ass – Arrogant and pretentious, translation of original phrase from the French *péter plus haut que son cul.*
Farthing – British coin currency with a nominal value. Benjamin Franklin uses the nominal currency as a double entendre at the end of his proposal to the Royal Academy of Brussels to create an award for an additive that word give farts a pleasant smell (see entry under Benjamin Franklin).
Farthingale – A hoop like structure worn under the skirt by women in the late 16th and early 17th centuries to give it the shape of a bell or cone. Originally introduced at the Spanish court it subsequently became popular fashion in Tudor England. Although the shape and structure may have been helpful to muffle the

sound and contain the aroma of a fart, there is no evidence that the name was related to the word fart. One theory behind the development of the farthingale was to hide a pregnancy that may have resulted from illicit relationships.

Fart in a bottle – Description of restless movement suggestive of agitation or being flustered.

Fart in a thunderstorm or windstorm –Figure of speech suggesting the event is unnoticed or unidentifiable because of background activity. When in the phrase as much chance as a fart in a thunderstorm, windstorm, blizzard, hurricane, tornado, gale, etc. it means having no chance at all.

Farting clapper - Anus, or more pejorative asshole.

Farting fanny – Nickname given to heavy German artillery guns used during World War I

Farting shot – An action designed to show contempt.

Farting through silk –financially affluent, able to afford luxuries

Fart lighting – Ignition of flammable gas (methane and/or hydrogen) released in some farts. Serious injury and burns have resulted from this activity, most often seen in adolescent males.

Fartman – A fictional superhero popularized by television and radio personality Howard Stern (see separate entry).

Fart monkey – Term of endearment, usually for a pet such as a dog or cat that farts whenever it needs to. The fart monkey can also serve as fart camouflage and be designated as the source of an errant fart.

Fart sucker – A parasite or toady willing to do whatever it takes to curry favor. Analogous to ass kisser, brown-nose equivalent. Interesting tie in to French slang for criminal suspect. The French pronounce suspect as soos-pay, the same way they would pronounce the words *sucé pet*, which translates literally as fart sucker. The French authorities can use the double entendre to express their dislike of a suspect without being chastised.

Fart time – Describes employed hours per week that fall between full-time and part-time employment. Usually defined as between 21 and 35 hours of work time per week.

Fire a stink torpedo - Fart
Fire the retro-rocket - Fart
Firing scud missiles - Fart
Fizzler - Fart
Flamethrower - Fart
Flamer - Fart
Flapper - Fart
Flatulate - Fart
Flatulence - Fart
Flatus - Fart
Flipper - Fart
Float an air biscuit - Fart
Floof - Fart
Fluffy - Fart

Fog slicer - Fart
Fowl howl - Fart
Fragrant fuzzy - Fart
Free-floating anal vapors - Fart
Free Jacuzzi - Fart
Freep - Fart
Frequency Actuated Rectal Tremor - Fart
Fumigate - Fart
Funky rollers - Fart
Gas attack - Fart
Gas blaster - Fart
Gas from the ass - Fart
Gas master - Fart
Gaseous intestinal by-products – Fart
Ghost turd - Fart
Grandpa - Fart
Gravy pants - Fart
Great brown cloud - Fart
Heinus anus - Fart
Hole flappage - Fart
Hole flapper - Fart
Honk - Fart
HUMrrhoids - Fart
Hydrogen bomb - Fart
Ignition - Fart
Insane in the methane - Fart
Invert a burp - Fart
Jet propulsion - Fart
Joan of Fart – Artful nickname for a female who has farted audibly or aromatically.
Jockey burner - Fart
Jumping guts - Fart
Just calling your name - Fart
Just keeping warm - Fart
Just the noise - Fart
Kaboom - Fart
K-Fart - Fart
Kill the canary - Fart
Lay a wind loaf - Fart
Lay an air biscuit - Fart
Leave a gas trap - Fart
Let a beefer - Fart
Let a brewer's fart – To have diarrhea.
Let each little bean be heard - Fart
Let one fly - Fart
Let one go - Fart
Let the beans out - Fart

Artsy Fartsy: Cultural History of the Fart Volume One

Lethal cloud - Fart
Letting one rip - Fart
Lingerer - Fart
Made a gas blast – Fart
Make a stink - Fart
Make a trumpet of one's ass – Fart
Mating call of the barking spider - Fart
Meteor – Fart
Methane bomb - Fart
Methane production experiment - Fart
Moon gas - Fart
Mud duck - Fart
Must be a sewer around - Fart
Nose death - Fart
Odor bubble - Fart
Odorama - Fart
Old fart – An old man, a person in authority very set in their ways, inflexible.
One-man jazz band - Fart
One-gun salute - Fart
Painting the elevator - Fart
Pant stainer - Fart
Panty burp - Fart
Parp - Fart
Party in your pants - Fart
Pass gas - Fart
Pass wind - Fart
Pet – Fart (French) The diminutive for fart in the French language. It makes the written English use of pet shop, pet food, love of pets, etc. an interesting translation. The pronunciation is different however, as pet is pronounced as pay in French
Pissed as a fart – Very drunk (British & Australian)
Play the tuba - Fart
Playing the trouser tuba - Fart
Plotcher (aka a wet one) – Fart
Poof - Fart
Poop gas - Fart
Poot - Fart
Pootie – Fart
Pop - Fart
Pop a fluffy - Fart
Preventing spontaneous human combustion – Fart
Puff, the magic dragon - Fart
Quack - Fart
Raspberry (Razz) - Slang for *'blowing a raspberry or strawberry'*, imitating the sound of a fart by exhaling through pursed lips, usually as a sign of derision. Also known as a Bronx cheer.

Rebuild the ozone layer one poof at a time - Fart
Rectal honk - Fart
Rectal shout - Fart
Rectal tremor - Fart
Release a squeaker - Fart
Release an ass biscuit - Fart
Release gas - Fart
Rep - Fart
Rimshot - Fart
Rip ass - Fart
Rip one - Fart
Ripple fart - Fart
Roast the Jockeys - Fart
Rotting vegetation - Fart
Royal fart – A fart of unusual distinction.
Safety - Fart
Salute your shorts - Fart
SAS (silent and scentless) – Fart
SBD (silent but deadly) – Fart
Set off an SBD - Fart
Shart – Fart passage that allows the escape of fecal material. The word shart is a portmanteau of shit and fart.
Shit fumes - Fart
Shit honker - Fart
Shit vapor - Fart
Shoot the cannon - Fart
Shoppin' at Wal-Fart - Fart
Silent and scentless (SAS) – Fart
Silent but deadly (SBD) – Fart
Singe the carpet - Fart
Singing the anal anthem - Fart
Sounding the sphincter scale - Fart
Sound of a barking spider - Fart
Sound of a wompus cat - Fart
Sparrow-fart - Denotes the earliest of daylight, early dawn, sunrise, sunup, first light of day.
Sphincter song - Fart
Spit a brick - Fart
Squeak one out - Fart
Squeaker - Fart
Steamer - Fart
Step on a duck - Fart
Step on a frog - Fart
Stink bomb - Fart
Stink burger - Fart

Strangling the stank monkey - Fart
Strawberry - Slang for imitating the sound of a fart by exhaling through pursed lips, usually as a sign of derision. Also known as a Bronx cheer.
Stress release - Fart
Tail wind - Fart
The colonic calliope - Fart
The dog did it - Fart
The F bomb - Fart
The gluteal tuba - Fart
The Sound and the Fury - Fart
The stink's gone into the fabric - Fart
The third state of matter - Fart
The toothless one speaks - Fart
Thunder pants - Fart
Thunderspray - Fart
Toilet tune - Fart
Toot - Fart
Toot your own horn - Fart
Trelblow - Fart
Triple flutter blast - Fart
Trouser cough - Fart
Trouser trumpet - Fart
Turd honking - Fart
Turd hooties - Fart
Turn on the air conditioning in the colon - Fart
Uncorked symphony - Fart
Under burp - Fart
Venting one - Fart
Wet one - Fart
What the dog did - Fart
Who Cut the Cheese - Fart
Wrong way burping - Fart
Zinger – Fart

X. Fart in Foreign Languages

American Sign Language:

The non-dominant hand is an "A" or an "S" handshape. The dominant hand is a bent hand and is held so that the fingers are underneath the pinkie side of the non-dominant "fist." The dominant hand "unbends" and bends one time as if showing gas escaping. Here is a "one handed" version of fart, both versions are widely used. You start by opening up the pinkie, and then the ring and middle finger. The index finger stays curled up. Then you reverse and close the middle, then ring, then pinkie fingers. For comic effect or emphasis you can puff one cheek and force a bit of air through your lips at the corner of your mouth.

Afrikaans: fart
Albanian: pordhÃ«, pjerdh; pordhë, hajvan, pjerdh
Arabic: ضرطة ,ضرط ,نفخة ضرط, ha ridge
Armenian: fart, basz toe
Avestan: pərəδaiti
Azerbaijani: osurmaq
Basque: fart
Belarusian: Ð¿ÐµÑ€Ð´ÐµÑ‚ÑŒ
Bulgaria: fart Флатуленция, пръдня
Catalan: pet, *colloq* pet, *colloq* torracollons, *colloq* tirar-se un pet, fer-se un pet
Chinese (Simplified): 屁, 放屁 屁 fom pee/ pie Chee
Chinese (Traditional): 屁, 放屁 屁 fom pee/ pie Chee
Croatian: prdnuti, vjetar, prdac, ispuštati vjetrove, prditi
Czech: prd
Danish: prut
Dutch: wind laten, winderigheid, een wind laten, een scheet laten, (slang) scheet (slang)
Esperanto: furzi, furzo
Estonian: pieru
Farsi: gooz bede, گوز، گوزیدن
Filipino: umut-ot, kabag-gas oh mo toot ka
Finnish: pieru
French: péter, pet, dis gas, péter (argot); lâcher une vesse; vesser pet (argot), vesse, merdeux
Galician: peidar
Georgian: fart
German: furz, flatulenz, fuhren sie gas, furzen, sich mit jedem dreck abgeben (Umgangsprache), scheißer (slang)
Greek: πέρδομαι (perdomai), ÎºÎ±Î½Ï‰, κλάνω, πέρδομαι κλανιά, πορδή
Haitian Creole: fart
Hebrew: "להפליץ", "נאד לתקוע (סלנג) נפיחה ,נאד (סלנג)
Hindi: पादना
Hmong: tso paus, tawb paus

Hungarian: fing, fingik, szellentés
Icelandic: rã¦fill
Ilokano: uttot
Indonesian: kentut
Irish: fart
Italian: fart, flatulenza, pass il gas, scoreggiare scoreggio, peto
Japanese: おなら, 屁, おならをする, 屁をこく（俗語） おなら, 屁（俗語）
Korean: 방귀뀌다, bung koo

Latin: pēdĕre
Latvian: fart
Lithuanian: bezdalius
Macedonia: Đ¿Ñ€Đ´ĐµĐ¶
Malay: kentut
Maltese: fart
Norwegian: fart
Persian: گوز, گوزیدن، گوز gooz bede
Philippine: kabag-gas, oh mo toot ka, umut-ot,
Polish: bpierd, pierdzieÄ‡, gazy jelitowe, parvee etra, vi pierdzieć, pierdnięcie, pierdnąć
Portugese: peidar, pedo, flatulência, soltar um pum (gíria) peido,
Romanian: bÄfÅŸi, flatulenţă, gaze (vulgar), vint, a da vinturi,

Russian: пердеть (perdet'), издавать громкий треск, пукнуть громкий треск при выходе газов из организма, непристойный звук; пукание; старик зря терять время Đ¿ĐµÑ€Đ´ĐµÑ‚ÑŒ, метеоризм, puk nee
The Russian words for fart include *perdyozh* (first act of breaking wind), *perdun* (perpetrator and outcome), *perdil'nik* (place from where it comes), *Perun* (ancient God of wind), *bzdun* (silent fart), *bzdyukha* (silent fart as well as a stupid jerk). Some of the Russian verbs for the action of farting are particularly colorful. *Perdet'* (to fart with or without sound), *bzdet'* (to fart silently), *pereperdet* (to fart repeatedly), and my favorite word *nabzdet'sya* (ton fart silently to one's complete and utter satisfaction!).

Sanskrit: pardate
Serbian: Đ¿Ñ€Đ´Ñ½ŃƒÑ‚Đ¸
Slovak: prd
Slovenian: prdec
Somali: doughso
Spanish: pedo, tirarse un pedo (familismo), peo, pasar gasses, peer, ventosear, ventoseo, cuesco
Swahili: fart, kyfoosi
Swedish: fart, fjärt , flatulens, prutta, fjärta (slang) prutt, fjärt (slang)
Tagalog (Philippine): kabag-gas, oh mo toot ka, umut-ot,
Taiwanese: 放屁 屁 funkee-pass gas
Thai: ตด, ฟาท, ลมตด (ผายลม),ตด,การผายลม,บตก,ผายลม
Turkish: osuruk, ul cer, osurmak, gaz yapmak osuruk, yellenme

Urdu: سڑنا باؤ -مارنا پھسکی یا پاد -پادنا ,گوز -باؤ -پھسکی -پاد ,گوز
Vietnamese: đánh rắm, trung tiện, dit, danh từ, đùi 0 rắm, nội động từ, chùi gháu
Visayan: otot
Welsh: basio gwynt
Yiddish: פֿאָרצן

XI. Afterword

Artsy Fartsy, Cultural History of the Fart is a fascinating and factually correct review of the common fart through human culture and history. It has a companion volume: ***To 'Air' is Human, Everything You Ever Wanted to Know About Intestinal Gas, which*** uniquely informative, entertaining, and well-illustrated. It covers everything you ever wanted to know about the fart, burp, and bloat but were too embarrassed to ask. Intestinal gas has been produced and released by virtually every human who has ever lived, yet very few people have been provided with the knowledge that can offer comfort and relief.

This volume is overflowing with practical information, fascinating facts, surprising trivia, and tasteful humorous insight about this universal phenomenon. Extensive knowledge about the physiology and science of the digestive process and intestinal gas is clearly explained. The knowledge gained will contribute to your enhanced health and comfort, and sharing this wisdom with others can leave a lasting impression on friends and family.

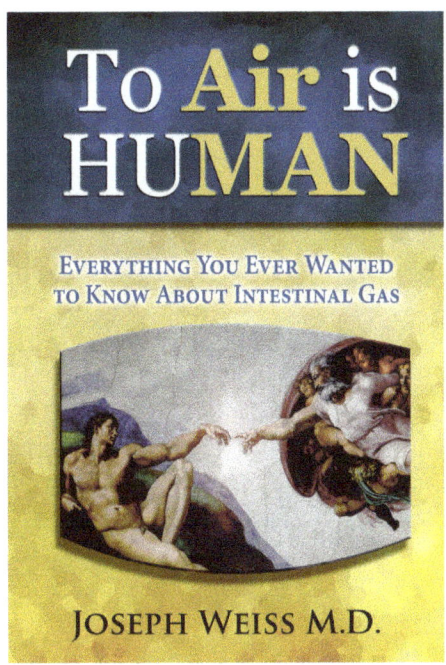
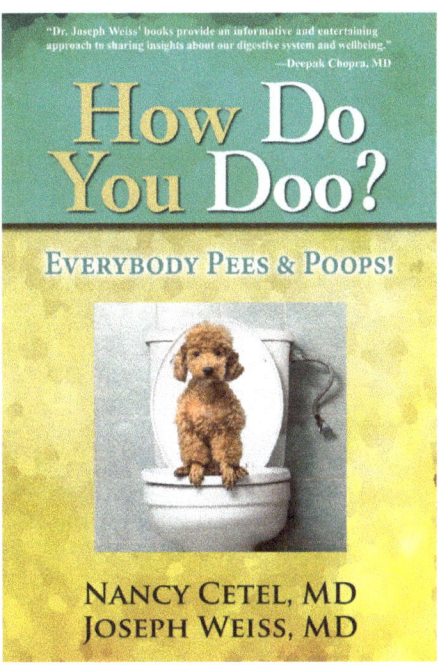

How Do You Doo? Everybody Pees & Poops! A delightfully informative, entertaining, and colorfully illustrated volume with valuable practical insights on toilet training. Tasteful color photographs of animals answering the call of nature allows the child to understand that everybody does it! Additional informative relevant content to entertain the adult while the child is 'on the potty' is included.

The Scoop on Poop! Flush with Knowledge is a uniquely informative tastefully entertaining, and well-illustrated volume that is full of it! The 'it' being a comprehensive and knowledgeable overview of all topics related to the remains of the digestive process. Whether you call it poop, feces, excrement, manure, dung, or the hundred plus other euphemisms, shit happens, and it happens a lot! Tens of billions of pounds and kilograms of it or deposited every day by while diversity of animal and microbial life. Humans alone contribute over three billion pounds a day, and only a small percentage of that is treated by a sewage system

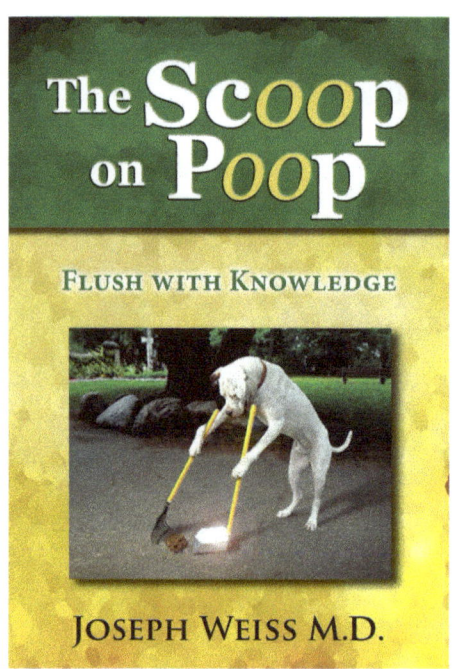
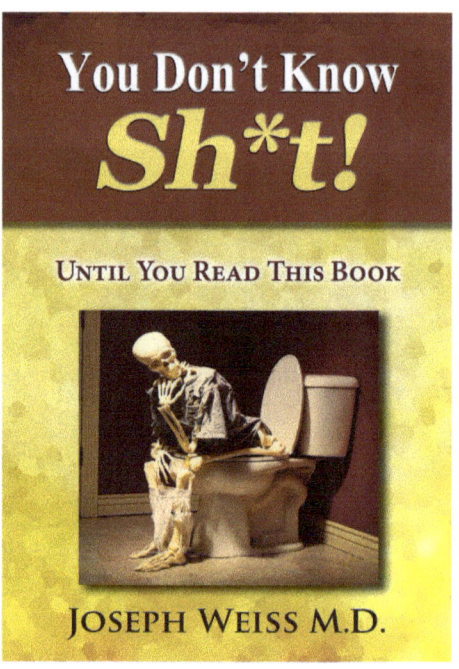

The identical content of The Scoop on Poop has been provocatively and cheekily retitled as ***You Don't Know Sh*t! Until You Read This Book***. This volume is an informative, entertaining and colorfully illustrated fountain of knowledge that is full of valuable information, including eccentricities and peculiarities, about the remains of the digestive process. Although this end result is politely described as feces or excrement, it is more commonly known by one of oldest words in the English language, shit. The book covers everything you ever wanted to know about this subject. Whether you disdain it, or appreciate it, it is part of the human (and animal) experience. The purpose of this volume is to share rarely discussed but very important knowledge about poop. The information ranges from the potentially life-saving to the sidesplitting descriptions of the eccentricities and peculiarities of human behavior on the subject matter. The wealth of information and trivia can sustain a long social conversation, or cut it short abruptly!

AirVeda: Ancient & New Medical Wisdom, Digestion & Gas covers the remarkable advances in the understanding of digestive health and wellness. New information about the critical role of genomics, epigenetics, the gut microbiome, and the gut-brain-microbiome-diet axis are opening new avenues to optimal whole body health and wellness. An appreciation of the ancient wisdom of Ayurveda and other disciplines shows that they had advanced insights into the nature of the human body and the holistic approach. Although intestinal gas, basic bodily functions, and feces have been topics culturally suppressed, knowledge and understanding are needed to achieve and maintain optimal health. This volume, and others in the series, provide an informative and entertaining in depth look at the amazing world of human health and digestion.

"Ayurveda is a 5,000 year old system of natural healing that reminds us that health is the balanced and dynamic integration between our environment, body, mind and spirit. In Dr. Joseph Weiss' book, AirVeda, he provides an informative and entertaining approach to sharing insights about our digestive system and wellbeing by applying the ancient wisdom of Ayurveda to everyday life." **Deepak Chopra, MD**

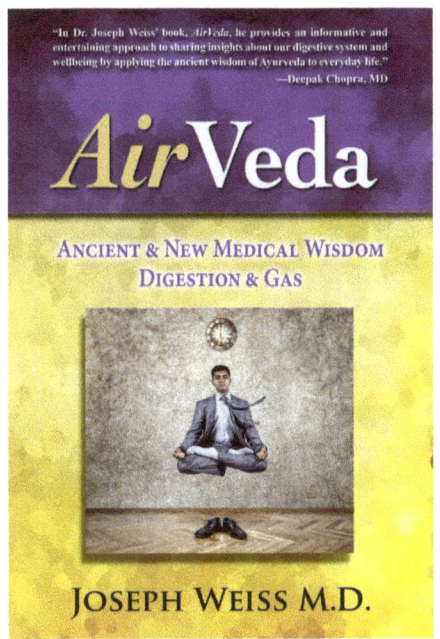
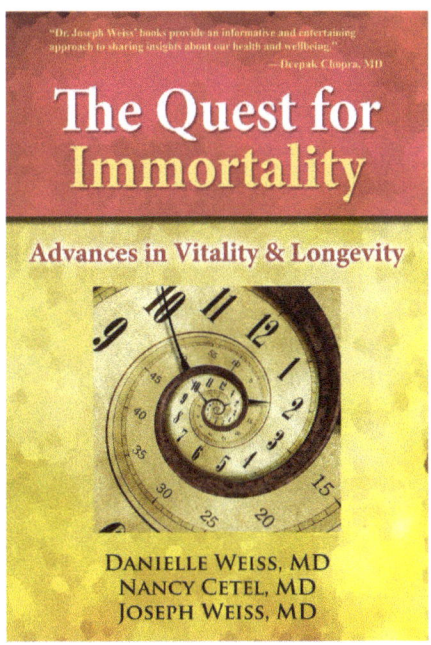

The Quest for Immortality, Advances in Vitality & Longevity provides an informative and enlightening overview of the remarkable advances in science and medicine that are dramatically enhancing human health and lifespan. The volume is written in clear, understandable, and engaging language with striking colorful illustrations. From groundbreaking nanotechnology to genomics and stem cells, the secrets of vitality and longevity are being uncovered along with more traditional advances and practical insights into disease prevention and health enhancement.

An even more comprehensive yet entertaining series are the extensive volumes of ***Digestive Health & Disease, An Illustrated Encyclopedia of Everything You Ever Wanted To Know About Digestion & Nutrition***. These volumes are a uniquely informative, entertaining, and lavishly illustrated compendium of alimentary knowledge and eccentricities. It covers everything you ever wanted to know about digestion and nutrition in health and disease. Volumes One through Five are available on Amazon.com.

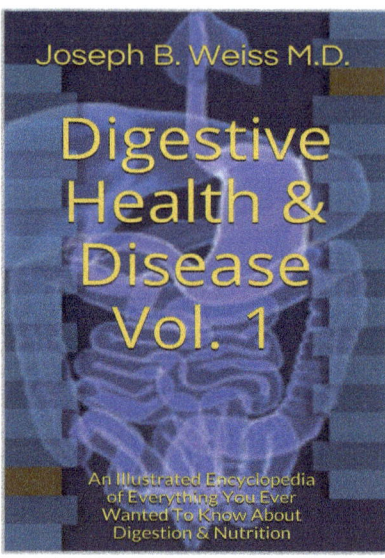 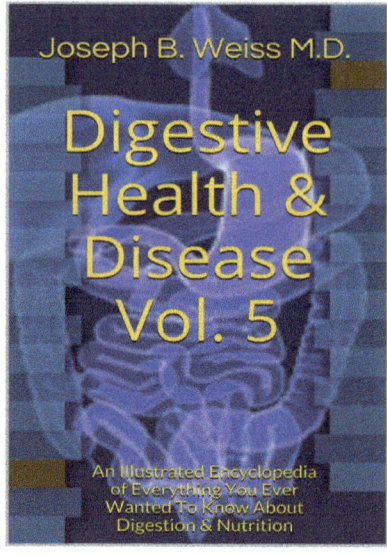

Organized as a reader friendly encyclopedia, the volumes cover over two thousand five hundred subject topics. Each volume may be utilized as an independent fully contained resource for the subjects it covers. The extensive size and scope of the series allows topics to be included that are rarely discussed in other books in the field and may be of great interest to the curious mind.

Written for the intelligent lay public, the medical and scientific terminology is translated into plain English. Practical and useful information and guidance are the primary goals, but entertaining and interesting information is included wherever possible. Designed for the visual learner as well, the clearly written text is supplemented by excellent photographs, illustrations, and charts. The reader will be informed, entertained, and the beneficiary of their newfound understanding of the universal process of digestion and metabolism that is the basis of all healthy living.

The website www.smartaskbooks.com has a complete list of books and programs by Joseph Weiss, MD, FACP, FACG, AGAF, Clinical Professor of Medicine (Gastroenterology), University of California, San Diego.

XII Index (including Volume Two)

Advertising & Marketing 65, 73-74, 75
Aerophagia 8
Afterword 185-188
Alighieri, Dante 177-178
Arabia, Lawrence of 143-144
Arabian Nights 135-138, 175-177
Aristophanes 171-173
Aristotle 88-90
Arouet, François-Marie (Voltaire) 204-207
Aubrey, John 197
Auden, W.H. 257-258
Augustine of Hippo (Saint Augustine) 108
Augustine, Saint 108
Babylonian Talmud 98-99
Balzac, Honoré 214-215
Banks, Iain 279-281
Barth, John 267-268
Baudelaire, Charles Pierre 219
Beardsley, Aubrey 51-53
Beavis & Butt-head 71
Bel-Phegor 82, 170
Beckett, Samuel 260-261
Bible Prophets 83
Blake, William 209-210
Blount, Thomas 126-127
Boilly, Louis-Léopold 28-29
Bollywood Hindi Movie 63
Bosch, Hieronymus 21-22
Bourke, John Gregory 138-140
Brillat-Savarin, Jean Anthelme 208-209
Bruegel the Elder, Pieter 24-25
Brooks, Mel 59-60
Budweiser Super Bowl Commercial 65
Burton, Sir Richard   135-138
Bush, George W. 159-160
Canadian Broadcast Corporation 57
Canterbury Tales 130-132
Carlin, George 272-275
Cartoonists 67-69
Chaucer, Geoffrey 180-182
Children's Book Art 69-70
Children's Books 284-288
Chronology of Farts in the Arts 21-81

Chronology of Farts in History 82-169
Chronology of Farts in Literature 170-288
Churchill, Sir Winston 144-147
Cicero 91-92
Cinematic Arts 59-63
Claudius 92-93
Clemens, Samuel (Mark Twain) 222-242
Colloquialism, Idiom, & Synonym of Fart 170-181
Commercial, Budweiser Super Bowl 49
Crepitation Contest 57
Cromwell, Oliver 121
Cruikshank, George 47-49
Cushion, Whoopee 100-101
Dahl, Roald 258-260
Dalai Lama of Tibet, H.H. the 14th 161-163
Dali, Salvador 57-59
Dante Alighieri 177-178
De Balzac, Honoré 153
Defoe, Daniel 197-199
De Gaulle, Charles 153-154
Dent, William 32
De Plancy, Jacques Collin 213-214
De Verville, Francois Béroalde 189-191
Digestion 7-20
di Lodovico Buonarroti Simoni, Michelangelo 23
Divine Comedy 177-178
Donne, John 193-194
Earl of Rochester, Lord John Wilmot 121-123, 199-200
Elagabalus 100
Elizabeth I, HRH Queen 115-117
Elizabeth II, H.M. Queen 155-156, 157-159
Ensor, James 55-57
Erasmus, Desiderius 111-112
Etymology - Origin of the Word Fart 4-6
Family Guy 71
Fart, Colloquialism, Idiom, & Synonym 170-181
Fart, Etymology (Word Origin) 5-7
Fart, Foreign Language 182-184
Fart, Physiology 7-20
Fielding, Henry 207-208
Flaubert, Gustave 220-222
Foreign Languages 182-184
Fox, Charles James 129-130
Franklin, Benjamin 123-126
Fraser, George MacDonald 266-267
Freud, Sigmund 140-143

Gaddafi, Muammar 160-161
Gillray, James 29-32
Global Warming 163-169
Goethe, Johann Wolfgang Von 211-213
Goya, Francisco 26-27
Hadith, Islam 109-110
Hemingway, Ernest 254-255
Herodotus 85-87
Heywood, John 184-185
Hippocrates 87-88
Hitler, Adolf 147-151
Hugo, Victor 216-218
Hutchinson, Sir Robert 152-153
Huxley, Aldous 249-252
Idioms 170-181
Index 189-193
Introduction 1-3
Islam Hadith 109-110
Japanese Lithographs Edo Period 35-47
Jerome, Saint 106-107
Jonson, Ben 191-193
Johnson, Lyndon Baines 154-155
Johnson, Samuel 182-183
Josephus, Flavius 95-96
Joyce, James 246-248
Kant, Immanuel 127-129
Kuniyoshi, Utagawa 35-47
Lama, HH Dalai 161-163
Langland, William 179-180
Lawrence, D.H. 248-249
Lawrence (of Arabia), T.E. 143-144
Lear, Edward 218-219
Le Pétomane 53-55
Lincoln, Abraham 131-134
Lion King 66
Lord John Wilmot, Earl of Rochester 121-123, 199-200
Ludlow, Henry 119-120
Luther, Martin 112-115
Mailer, Norman 263-264
Marchetta, Melina 282-283
Marketing & Advertising 65, 73-81
Martialis, Marcus Valerius 174-175
Medieval Manuscripts 24-26
Metrocles 90
Michelangelo di Lodovico Buonarroti Simoni 23
Miller, Henry 253-254

Miller's Tale 180-182
Milton, John 195-196
Montaigne, Michel de 117-118
Moore, Sir Thomas 110-111
Mozart, Wolfgang Amadeus 27-29
Movies 59-63
Mr. Methane 64-65, 77
Nesbø, Jo 288
Newton, Richard 34
Oldfield, Paul 64-61
Ontario Ministry of Health 73-74
Patterson, James 277-279
Peasant's Fart 178-179
Petronius 173-174
Physiology – Digestion and the Fart 7-20
Piers Plowman 179-180
Plutarch   97-98
Preface VIII-IX
Prince Philip, HRH 157-158
Prophets, Bible 83
Pujol, Joseph 53-55
Pythagoras 83-84
Queen Elizabeth I, H.M 115-117
Queen Elizabeth II, H.M. 155-156, 157-159
Rabelais, François 182-184
Reagan, Ronald 155-157
Rochester, Earl of, Lord John Wilmot 90, 143
Roth, Philip 270--272
Rushdie, Salman 275-277
Rutebeuf 178-179
Saint Augustine 108
Saint Jerome 106-107
Salinger, J.D. 261-262
Seinfeld 64
Seneca 93-95
Shakespeare, William 185-189
Simpsons 71
Sir Richard Burton 135-137, 126
Sir Winston Churchill 144-147
Sir Robert Hutchinson 146-147
Sir Thomas Moore 110-111
Sir Salman Rushdie 275-277
Sir John Suckling 194-195
South Park 71
Stalin, Josef 151-152
Stern, Howard 281-282

Stoutshanks, S. 50
Styron, William 264-265
Suckling, Sir John 194-195
Super Bowl Budweiser Commercial 49
Swift, Jonathon 200-203
Synonyms 289-300
Talmud, Babylonian 98-99
Tales of Gargantua and Pantagruel 182-184
Tibet, H.H. the 14th Dalai Lama 161-163
Toole, John Kennedy 268-269
Twain, Mark (Samuel Clemens) 222-242
Voltaire (François-Marie Arouet) 204-207
Von Goethe, Johann Wolfgang 28, 151-152
Vonnegut, Jr., Kurt 262-263
Wagner, Richard 50-51
Warming, Global 115-120
Wells, William 33
Wenling, Chen 72-73
Whoopee Cushion 100-101
Wilmot, Lord John, Earl of Rochester 121-123, 199-200
Wolfe, Thomas 255-257
Yoga 101-106
Zola, Émile 242-246

www.ingramcontent.com/pod-product-compliance
Lightning Source LLC
Chambersburg PA
CBHW040221040426
42333CB00049B/3061